Praise for Dave Zinczenko's
Eat This, Not That!

"Will freak the weight right off of you!"
—ELLEN DEGENERES

Praise for *Eat It to Beat It!*

"David Zinczenko's investigations into the truth about our food make him one of the top nutrition experts in America. Eat It to Beat It! is an essential guidebook for anyone with an appetite for eating and living well."
—TRAVIS STORK, M.D.
Co-host, *The Doctors*

Also by David Zinczenko

Banish Belly Fat—and Take Back Your Health—While Eating the Brand-Name Foods You Love!

EAT IT TO BEAT IT!

DAVID ZINCZENKO

BALLANTINE BOOKS TRADE PAPERBACKS • NEW YORK

No book can replace the diagnostic expertise and medical advice of a trusted physician. Please be certain to consult with your doctor before making any decisions that affect your health, particularly if you suffer from any medical condition or have any symptom that may require treatment.

A Ballantine Books Trade Paperback Original

Published in the United States by Ballantine Books, an imprint of Random House, a division of Random House LLC, a Penguin Random House Company, New York.

BALLANTINE and the HOUSE colophon are registered trademarks of Random House LLC.

ISBN 978-0-345-54793-4
eBook ISBN 978-0-345-54794-1

Printed in the United States of America on acid-free paper

www.ballantinebooks.com

9 8 7 6 5 4 3 2 1

Design by George Karabotsos, with Laura White.
Photos by Daniel Egongoro. Photo direction by Tara Long.

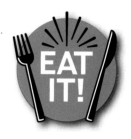

DEDICATION

To everyone working to protect their
well-being and that of their families.
May this book be an essential weapon
in your health and happiness arsenal.

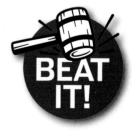

ACKNOWLEDGMENTS

This book would not have been possible without the support, guidance, and hard work of the following:

Gina Centrello, Bill Takes, Libby Mcguire, Marnie Cochran, Jennie Tung, Richard Callison, Joe Perez, Nina Shield, Susan Corcoran, Theresa Zoro, Cindy Murray, Sanyu Dillon, Kristin Fassler, and Quinne Rogers at Ballantine.

Stephen Perrine, publisher and chief creative officer, and George Karabotsos, design director, of Galvanized.

Heather Hurlock, master of food intelligence gathering, and Tara Long, who shopped and styled these pages.

Steve Gilbert, Ray Jobst, Jon Hammond, Allison Zinczenko, Charlene Lutz, and the Galvanized team.

Sara Vigneri, Daniel Engongoro, Ashley Ross, Amelia Harnish, Laura White, Peter Yang, Wendy Hess, and many others who contributed to this effort.

Ben Sherwood, Robin Roberts, George Stephanopoulos, Sam Champion, Barbara Fadida, Lara Spencer, Josh Elliot, and the team at *Good Morning America,* whose support has been critical to launching this franchise.

Jennifer Rudolph Walsh, Jon Rosen, Andy McNichol, and the brilliant minds at WME.

Larry Shire, Eric Sacks, and Jonathan Ehrlich, for their invaluable counsel.

Mehmet Oz, Travis Stork, David Pecker, Strauss Zelnick, Joe Armstrong, Dan Abrams, and the many friends, colleagues, and advisors who continue to inspire me with their wisdom and insight.

And to the best family a man could be blessed with.

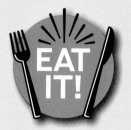

EAT IT!

EAT IT TO BEAT IT!

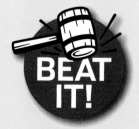

BEAT IT!

CONTENTS

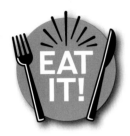

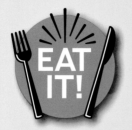

EAT IT TO BEAT IT!

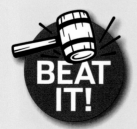

OUR FOOD UNDER ATTACK

Hi, folks! Thanks for dining with us tonight!

We've got some delicious specials for you. Our featured pizza comes on a dough built partially from plastic foam, topped with additives made from human hair, duck feathers, and the desiccated abdomens of beetles, and finished with a delicate dusting of silicon dioxide—you know it as sand. And for the kids, we have a yummy selection of ice creams blended with wood shavings and flavored with extract from the anal scent glands of beavers. And as always, your meal comes free with a chef's selection of more than half a dozen chemicals that are only suspected of causing—but let me emphasize, have not yet been 100 percent proven to cause—obesity, hyperactivity, asthma, cancer, and diabetes!

Wait, can this all be true? Are we feeding our kids anal scent glands and human hair? Yes, in fact, as well as more than 3,000 natural and artificial chemicals approved by the Food and Drug Administration as preservatives, additives, and artificial and "natural" flavorings. (Wood chips, beaver anuses, and beetle bellies are natural, so they're among the "natural" ingredients you might be enjoying tonight.)

So if you're wondering why watching your weight has become so challenging—why all the diet foods and the low-carb this and low-fat that aren't making a difference—it might have to do with something more than your willpower. It might have to do with the fact that much of the food we're buying is filled with things that only vaguely qualify as "food," and that marketers and manufacturers are using a remarkable array of tricks, tools, and tactics to fool us into buying their products.

In fact, as more and more Americans become health-conscious—as we spend more time reading labels and looking for "whole foods," "organic foods," and "natural foods" (not to mention gluten-free, vegan, non-GMO, unsweetened, low-fat, dairy-free, no-high-fructose-corn-syrup-added foods), marketers have become even more savvy at finding ways to force-feed us things that can make us fat, without our even knowing.

You can follow any diet plan out there, but unless you know exactly what's in your food, no diet is really going to make a difference.

Not until you learn how to *Eat It to Beat It!*

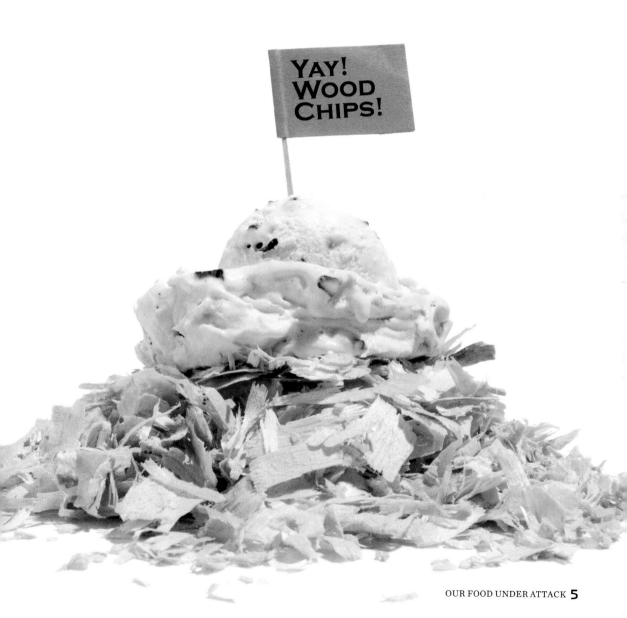

YAY!
WOOD
CHIPS!

WHY IS OUR FOOD SO WEIRD?

As I said, there are more than 3,000 food additives approved by the FDA, and all of them have been proven safe for humans.

No, wait . . . that's not exactly true. Of those 3,000 chemicals, the FDA only has chemical and "administrative" information on about one third of them. On the remaining 2,000, the administration claims to have chemical and toxicological information, including substances considered "generally recognized as safe," or GRAS. And worst of all, they admit that their 3,000-additive list, titled "Everything Added to Food in the United States," is only a partial list because manufacturers can add things to food that they themselves deem to be GRAS. Yes, you read that right: Manufacturers can just tell the FDA that a substance they're using meets the GRAS standards.

And that's too bad, because like you, I love junk food. Unlike most healthy-eating advocates, I'm not all about forsaking fries and Fudgsicles for falafel and fruit salad.

But what's happened is that food marketers have taken good old-fashioned bad-for-us food and turned it into crazy science-fiction food. They're taking all the good clean fun out of eating bad! For example, if you regularly enjoy frozen desserts and shredded cheeses, check the label; it may list an ingredient called "cellulose," which is, in fact, shredded wood chips! I want ice cream, chocolate fudge, gooey cookies, crunchy fries, creamy shakes. But I don't want the food industry dumping weird chemicals into them.

And if you don't think all these crazy additives and preservatives are having an impact on your weight, think again. For example, let's say you wanted to make something called an Oreo sundae. What would you do? Get some vanilla ice cream, crush some Oreos, pour some chocolate syrup on it, and presto: A totally indulgent, bad-for-you dessert. A ½ cup of Edy's vanilla topped with 2 tbsp of Hershey's chocolate syrup and a couple of Oreo cookies will cost you 400 calories, most of it from fat and sugar. But hey, ya gotta live, right?

But here's where eating bad turns into eating horrible: What happens if you go to a Baskin-Robbins and order their Oreo Layered Sundae? Things get a little more "evil genius" than they do in your own kitchen. The folks at Baskin-Robbins somehow created a science experiment with 79 ingredients—11 of which are some form of sugar. As a result, you're downing 1,330 calories—more than three times what you'd eat if you just made it at home.

Just take a look at how catastrophically caloric our restaurant meals have gotten. In a recent study in the *Journal of the American Medical Association,* researchers looked at 19 chain restaurants, studying a typical breakfast, lunch, and dinner. Their findings were pretty stunning. The average restaurant meal contains:

1,128 calories, or about 56 percent of a person's daily calorie intake.

2,269 milligrams of sodium, or 95 percent of a person's daily recommended intake. (In fact, researchers consider 600 milligrams or less a "healthy" meal, yet only 1 percent of all chain restaurant meals meet this standard!)

58 grams of fat (89 percent of what we should eat in a day.)

And things aren't any better in the supermarket aisles, either! In the dessert section, Pepperidge Farms 3-Layer Coconut Cake boasts 32 ingredients, including propylene glycol (an ingredient in antifreeze). In the chips and dips aisle, Pace Jalapeno and Pepper Jack Dip has 53 ingredients, and salt is listed six times. And in the freezer compartment, Tombstone Deep Dish Pepperoni and Cheese Supreme clocks in with 116 ingredients, including L-cysteine listed three times. What's L-cysteine? A dough conditioner derived from natural sources, the most common of which is human hair or poultry feathers. It's also got some partially hydrogenated oils (artery-clogging trans fats), BHT (a component of embalming fluid), and "Natural flavor," which can include any number of bizarre organic ingredients, including the above-mentioned beaver anus.

What makes our food that much more troubling is that there are so many technical terms at play that it's hard for anyone, even the manufacturers themselves, to really know what's in the product. "Natural and artificial flavors," for example, are proprietary concoctions that food marketers buy from big chemical companies to add to their food. Meanwhile, ingredient labels are starting to look more and more like Tolstoy novels, reaching such overwhelming length that nobody has time to read them anymore. Nowadays you'll find products that list things like corn syrup, molasses, dextrose, sucrose, brown rice syrup, and cane invert syrup, all on the same package. Except that every single one of those things can be called by another name: sugar. Same for things like sodium: Sodium nitrate, sodium diacetate, sodium phosphate, sodium erythorbate, and other forms can all show up on the same side label, confounding your attempts to cut down on "salt." As a result, the average American man now eats, *every single day:*

²/₃ cup of sugar
½ cup of fats and shortenings
2 teaspoons of salt
500 calories more than he burns off

Is it any surprise, then, that we spend nearly $200 a year per person—man, woman, and child—in America on prescription drugs to fight diabetes, high blood pressure, and cholesterol?

Do you think there might be a better way? I do.

THE NEW NUTRITION FRONT

Back in 2007, when I wrote the first in a series of Eat This, Not That! books, I was on a mission: to get restaurants and food manufacturers to start giving us honest, accessible information on how many calories they were serving us—and how much fat and sodium as well.

Maybe it was my own lifelong struggles with weight that motivated me. As a teenager growing up in a single-parent household, I was left to fend for myself a lot, nutritionally. Fast food was my go-to lunch and dinner, and "home cooking" was anything out of a box, bag, or can. By age 14, I weighed more than 200 pounds. I was such a languid lump of loaming that the high school wrestling coach recruited me, literally, to sit on people. And when I started my career in health journalism, I was self-conscious about my weight; how was I supposed to help advise others when I was carrying a history of junk food under my belt—literally?

That's where my quest to understand nutrition began. I started looking into what was really in our food, and how much fat, sugar, and calories we were eating, especially at our favorite restaurants.

Back then, very few restaurants gave consumers access to nutritional information, and when I began calling them out on their outrageously fat-, sugar-, and calorie-loaded foods, many threatened to sue.

But in the end, the food manufacturers began to see the light. They began posting nutrition information on their menus and on their websites, and several municipalities began requiring calorie counts from major chains. And as a result—well, we might just be making some progress. In the summer of 2013, for the first time since government agencies have tracked these trends, the Centers for Disease Control reported a decline in childhood obesity among underprivileged kids, our most vulnerable population group. Nineteen states, from Georgia to New Jersey to California, showed measurable declines; the vast majority of other states showed no increase, after decades of rising obesity rates.

But the more you study nutrition—especially when it comes to the devious, dissembling double-talk on our food packaging and restaurant menus—the more you realize that calories alone aren't the whole story. According to data collected by the CDC, Americans now get 70 percent of their calories from processed food. If you want to control you weight, your health, and your life, you need to understand what, exactly, is in the foods you're eating.

And this book is the next step in taking control.

WHAT DID YOU JUST PUT IN YOUR MOUTH?

According to the National Institutes of Health, here's what we eat the most of as a nation, in terms of calories spent:

#1 Bread
#2 Cakes and Cookies
#3 Soda
#4 Alcohol
#5 Beef

Leaving aside the booze for now, if we could eat healthier versions of the other four, we'd be making huge strides toward living leaner, longer, and better. Let's break down the trouble spots.

BREAD. Most of the bread we eat today is made from enriched flour and high-fructose corn syrup, and even much of what is sold as "wheat bread" isn't actually whole grain. Worse, many commercial breads contain cellulose (that's the wood pulp I was talking about), as well as azodicarbonamide, a foaming agent also found in yoga mats and the heels of your running shoes.
EAT IT TO BEAT IT! Lower your risk of weight gain and discover the brands of bread that can help strip away the pounds on page 52.

CAKES AND COOKIES. You know they're going to have plenty of fat and sugar, but you need to indulge your tastebuds now and then, right? Problem is, you're often getting a heaping dose of something more troublesome than just fat and sugar: trans fats. The American Heart Association recommends keeping trans fats to just 1 percent of our daily calories, or no more than about 2 grams a day. But eat one of Marie Callender's Small Apple Pies and you'll get 12 grams of the stuff—about 108 calories' worth.
EAT IT TO BEAT IT! Reduce your risk of heart disease by discovering the healthiest, most delicious desserts in the supermarket and in all your favorite restaurants on page 84.

SODA. Why does it rank so high? Because of all the sugar. Mountain Dew, for example, not only delivers 52 grams of sugar per 12-ounce can, but it also gives you a delicious side helping of bromated vegetable oil, a component of rocket fuel. And I don't mean metaphorical rocket fuel—I mean the actual stuff they put in engines to keep the gears from exploding.
EAT IT TO BEAT IT! Cut diabetes out of your destiny by learning to drink right on page 272.

BEEF. It's not the beef that you should have a beef with, it's all the crazy sauces and toppings it often comes with. Many chain restaurants have steak and burger options that top 1,800 calories each—meaning one meal that has as many calories as a woman should eat in a whole day. Yet there are plenty of healthy options at places like Outback, Uno Chicago Grill, and TGI Friday's.
EAT IT TO BEAT IT! Indulge your meat cravings while stripping away dozens of pounds from your midsection on pages 78, 102, and 288.

You don't need to spend a fortune in health-food stores, and you don't need to subsist on a diet of tofu and teff, to start losing weight fast and finding your path back to optimum health. I found hundreds of delicious foods in every category, from pizza to chocolate, from hamburgers to French fries, from yogurt to pasta, that are actually healthy for you. And these foods are found in your local supermarket and in your favorite chain restaurant.

The products you'll find recommended in *Eat It to Beat It!* have been studied, compared, and, in some cases, their manufacturers interrogated to ascertain just how healthy they are. I've eliminated the versions that are loaded with unnecessary junk (trust me, you won't miss the azodicarbonamide flavor at all).

So grab a fork, and start indulging your way back to health!

WHAT WE REALLY EAT— AND WHAT IT REALLY DOES TO US

		The Average Man age 20-49	The Average Woman* age 20-49
WE EAT TOO MUCH			
CALORIES	Should Be:	2,200	1,800
	Actually Is:	2,697	1,858
SUGAR	Should Be:	9 tsp	6 tsp
	Actually Is:	31 tsp	25 tsp
FAT	Should Be:	65 g	65 g
	Actually Is:	93.3 g	66 g
SODIUM	Should Be:	2,400 mg	2,400 mg
	Actually Is:	4,243 mg	2,980 mg
WE EAT TOO LITTLE			
VITAMIN E	Should Be:	15 mg	15 mg
	Actually Is:	8.9 mg	7.1 mg
VITAMIN D	Should Be:	15 mcg	15 mcg
	Actually Is:	5.9 mcg	4.5 mcg
VITAMIN A	Should Be:	900 mcg	700 mcg
	Actually Is:	682 mcg	60 mcg
FIBER	Should Be:	38 g	25 g
	Actually Is:	18.7 g	15.5 g
WE PAY THE PRICE			
Average # of Prescription Drugs Currently Used		3.7	4.2

*The Centers for Disease Control and Prevention report that American women, over time, average close to an appropriate daily calorie intake. But obesity rates among women are still incredibly high, in part because of yo-yo diet trends, and in part because of the effects of processed foods. That's why this book should become an essential part of your health-management plan."

⅔ cup of sugar!

nearly ½ cup of shortening!

a Tbsp of salt!

MONEY SPENT YEARLY (per person) ON PRESCRIPTIONS FOR

Diabetes	$79.24
Cholesterol	$66.13
High blood pressure	$47.61
Depression	$34.71
All other illnesses	$411.97

YOUR EDIBLE CHEMISTRY SET

Do you have any idea what you put in your mouth today?

"Of course," you say. "An Egg McMuffin, a pack of Twizzlers, a can of Sierra Mist, a turkey sandwich . . ."

Well, that's what those things were called. But what were they actually made out of?

The fact is, almost none of us has any idea what's really going into our food. Additives and preservatives derived from duck feathers, petroleum products, and even human hair make it impossible to control our food intake, unless we hunt, kill, and cook every meal ourselves. Today our food supply is a complicated chemistry set of organic and synthetic compounds, many of them listed under arcane phrases like "natural color" or "artificial flavor" that tell us nothing of what's going into our bodies.

For example, few vegetarians actually eat vegetarian on any given day. (As an example, the first food listed here would seem to fit into a vegetarian's diet, if it weren't for the dead beavers . . . as you'll see.) And anybody who thinks they're following a Paleo diet had better be dragging elk into their caves themselves, because many of our prepackaged meat and vegetable products are filled with post-industrial-revolution inventions.

To give you an idea of just how hard it is to know what we're eating, I took four common foods—stuff you see in supermarkets and chain restaurants every day—and listed their ingredients, alphabetically. All you have to do is read the ingredients list, and tell me what the food is. Don't worry about getting the exact product right. Just see if you can figure out in what aisle of the supermarket or what section of the menu this "food" would appear.

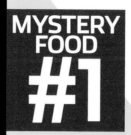

MYSTERY FOOD #1

Ingredients (in alphabetical order):

Almond butter
Ascorbic acid
Brown rice flour
Calcium phosphate
Canola oil
Dextrose ——————— *A form of sugar*
Ferrous fumarate
Fructose ——————————— *A form of sugar*
Maltodextrin ————————— *A form of sugar*
Milled rice
Natural flavor — *"Natural flavor" is a cocktail that can include a whole host of unknowns, including castoreum made from the glandular juice of beaver anus. It is a common source of vanilla flavoring.*
Nonfat milk
Oat bran
Organic evaporated cane juice syrup
————————— *A form of sugar*
Peanut flour
Potassium phosphate
Riboflavin
Rice bran
Rosemary extract
Salt
Soy lecithin
Soy protein isolate
Thiamine mononitrate
Vegetable glycerin
Vitamin B6 hydrochloride

HINT:
This is marketed as a health food for people who want "optimum performance."

Mystery item revealed on next page

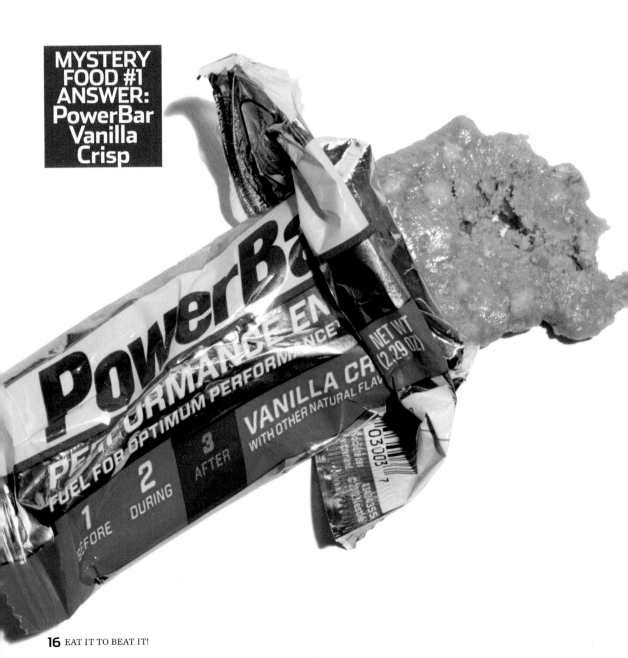

I'm a fan of well-chosen energy bars as a snack, protein source, or pre- or post-workout treat. That said, this one fails the "bar" by containing 5 different forms of sugar—for a total of 26 grams when you should try to get under 20; just one measly gram of fiber—when you should be getting at least three. To read how to choose a better version, see page 204.

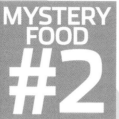

MYSTERY
FOOD
#2

Ingredients (in alphabetical order):

Artificial flavors — *Meaning, a flavor compound not found in products intended for human consumption*

Carrageenan

Cellulose gel

Cellulose gum — *Cellulose is wood chips "digested" with chemicals*

Citric acid

Cocoa

Confectioner's corn flakes

Cornstarch

Corn syrup

Cream

Ground roasted peanuts

Hydrogenated palm kernel oil — *A source of trans fats*

Lactic acid esters

Locust bean gum

Mono and diglycerides

Molasses *Originally derived from coal tar, this coloring is now mostly derived from petroleum*

Nonfat milk (twice)

Red 40

Salt

Soybean oil

Soy lecithin

Sugar (twice)

TBHQ — *Used to preserve freshness, it's also used as a corrosion inhibitor in biodiesel*

Vanilla extract

Vitamin A palmitate

Whey

Whey powder

Yellow 5

HINT:
Buy a "mini" for your four-year-old and she'll get 430 calories and 54 grams of sugar. Buy a large for yourself and enjoy 1,150 calories and 141 grams of sugar—the equivalent of 5 Butterfinger candy bars.

Mystery item revealed on next page

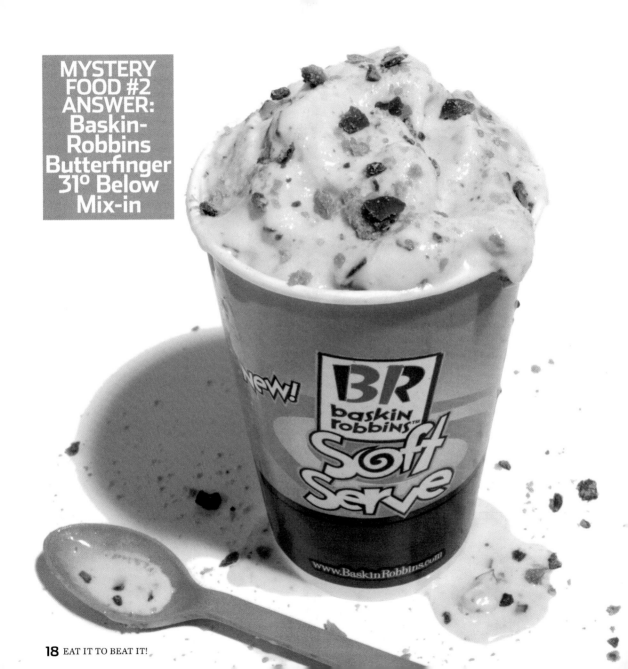

Life isn't much fun if you can't indulge in delicious desserts. But order the large and you're getting three meals' worth of this treat, plus wood chips, artificial flavors, a bit of Red 40 coloring, 35 teaspoons of sugar, and 130 percent of your recommended daily allowance of saturated fat. Does Baskin-Robbins really need to offer an ice cream treat with more calories than two Big Macs?

MYSTERY FOOD #3

Ingredients (in alphabetical order):

Ammonium sulfate
Annatto
Artificial butter flavor
Artificial flavor (listed twice)
Ascorbic acid
Azidocarbonamide
Barley malt
Beta carotene
Calcium peroxide
Calcium phosphate
Calcium propionate
Calcium sulfate
Cheese cultures
Citric acid (2 times)
Coarse ground pepper
Coloring
Corn flour
Dry cream
Egg whites
Egg yolks
Enzymes (listed twice)
Folic acid
High fructose corn syrup
Iron
L-cysteine
Medium chain triglycerides
Milk
Milkfat

Modified corn starch
Mono and diglycerides
Monocalcium phosphate
Natural flavor (listed twice)
Niacin
Oleoresin paprika color
Palm oil
Pork
Potassium sorbate
Propylene glycol
Riboflavin
Salt (listed 5 times)
Smoke flavoring
Sodium citrate
Sodium erythorbate
Sodium phosphate
Sodium nitrite
Sodium stearoyl lactylate
Sorbic acid
Soy lecithin (listed 3 times)
Soybean oil (listed 3 times)
Spice
Sugar
TBHQ
Thiamine mononitrate
Water (listed 4 times)
Wheat flour
Wheat gluten
Xantham gum
Yeast

Also used to make yoga mats

A component in anti-freeze

All forms of salt

The most common source of this chemical: human hair

HINT:
Start your morning with a coffee and one of these babies, and you'll get 57 percent of your sodium intake and half your saturated fat allowance just at breakfast!

Mystery item revealed on next page

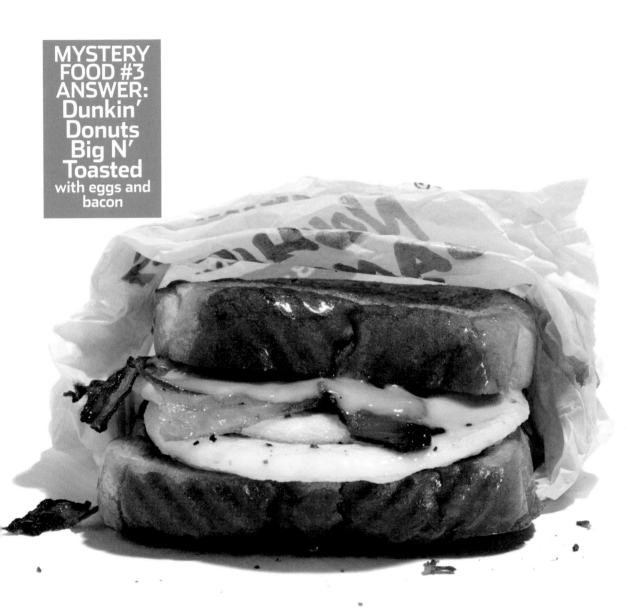

MYSTERY
FOOD #3
ANSWER:
Dunkin'
Donuts
Big N'
Toasted
with eggs and
bacon

Sure, it's a sandwich, so the ingredients list will always be a little long. But consider that the "fried eggs" portion of the sandwich has 13 ingredients alone, including stuff Grandma never put on her griddle: propolyne glycol, medium chain tryglycerides, and modified corn starch among them. And is there a reason why the bread, the eggs, the bacon and the cheese all have water as an ingredient?

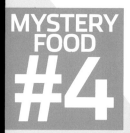

MYSTERY FOOD #4

Ingredients (in alphabetical order):

Autolyzed yeast extract (twice) — A source of MSG
BHT
Bleached wheat flour
Chicken breast with rib meat
Cornstarch
Dextrose — A form of sugar
Extractives of paprika
Flavoring
Garlic powder
Guar gum
Monocalcium phosphate
Salt (three times)
Sodium acid pyrophosphate
Sodium bicarbonate — Allows meat to retain water. Also used to get stains out of leather
Sodium tripolyphosphate
Soybean oil
Soy protein isolate
Spices — Concentrated soy mimicks the effects of estrogen
Sugar
Textured soy protein concentrate
Vegetable oil
Water (twice)
Yeast
Yellow corn flour

HINT: *This comes in a resealable family pack!*

Mystery item revealed on next page

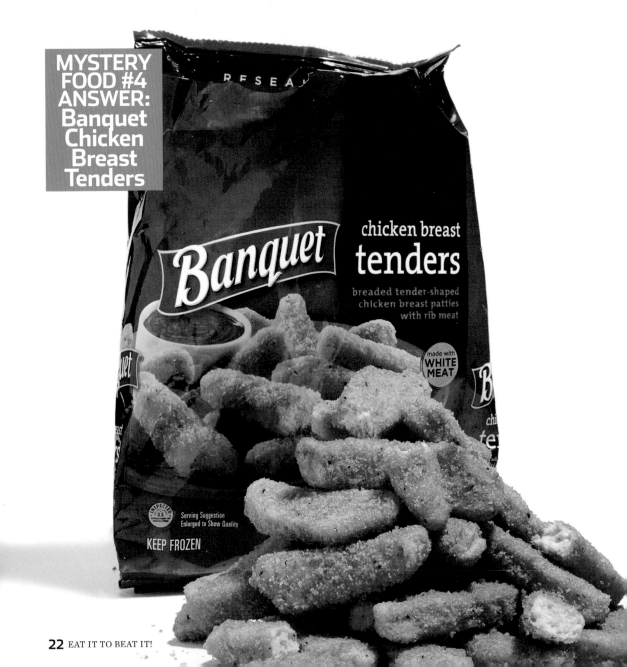

MYSTERY
FOOD #4
ANSWER:
Banquet
Chicken
Breast
Tenders

RESEAR

Banquet

chicken breast
tenders

breaded tender-shaped
chicken breast patties
with rib meat

made with
**WHITE
MEAT**

Serving Suggestion
Enlarged to Show Quality

KEEP FROZEN

If you guessed, "Some kind of meat," you're close enough! What happened to chicken breast tenders made with chicken, egg, buttermilk, flour, oil, and a bit of seasoning? Unfortunately, this kind of complexity is standard for foods in the freezer section.

HOW THIS BOOK WILL HELP YOU LOSE WEIGHT, FEEL GREAT, AND LIVE BETTER THAN EVER!

CHAPTER 1

Here's the dirty little secret the diet industry doesn't want you to know: Losing weight is much easier than you think.

I know, I know: If you've watched the afternoon talk shows or the late-night infomercials, visited a gym, or checked out a weight-loss website, then you've received thousands of messages about how you need to cut out fat, I mean carbs, I mean dairy, I mean gluten; about how you need to work out with Zumba, I mean Crossfit, I mean P90X, I mean Bowflex; about how you need to eat for your blood type, I mean pH level, I mean body composition, I mean astrological sign. Things have gotten so bizarre that there's now a program called the K-E Diet in which you take in all your food through a tube going up your nose.

All of this confusion is not helping.

While exercise is great, in any form, weight loss is primarily a matter of eating food that's good for you—and not too much of it. (And never up your nose.) And theoretically, that ought to be easy: When you cut 3,500 calories (or use them up with exercise) you lose a pound of weight. So, when your body is receiving the proper level of nutrients and the proper number of calories, in most cases your weight drops to its healthy, natural state and stays there. The more fit and active you are, the more calories you can take in and burn off.

So what's with all the craziness? Why are two out of every three Americas overweight or obese? Why does diabetes—once a condition of the wealthy and overfed—now eat up one in every five of our health care dollars? Why are so many of our toddlers ready to topple over?

It's primarily because the food we eat just isn't good for us.

And that's why I believe this book is truly revolutionary.

THE REAL WAY TO EAT SMART

While calories are a critical part of any nutrition plan, they're not the whole story. You can cut calories all you want and still find yourself eating a diet packed with sugar, salt, fat, and disease-causing additives that can play havoc with your weight and your health.

So when it came time to assess the most popular foods in America, I didn't just look at calorie counts. I took a deeper dive into the ingredients lists, keeping in mind that foods with seemingly believable health claims—even those that are low in calories, sodium, and the like—often hide nutritional subterfuge that undermines all the good a food might advertise on its front label.

Consider all the hype about yogurt. A 2012 study in the *International Journal of Obesity* found that dieters who ate three servings of fat-free yogurt a day lost 22 percent more weight and 61 percent more body fat than those who skipped the yogurt. The source of yogurt's power is its high level of protein and relatively low sugar. At just 100 calories, Siggi's Icelandic Style Skyr Non Fat Vanilla gives you a whopping 14 grams of belly-filling protein and just 9 grams of sugar. But over at Stonyfield Farm Organic, their Vanilla Over Chocolate gives you only half as much protein and 34 grams of sugar—as much as you'll find in 6 Chips Ahoy! Chewy cookies. That's not a food that should appear as a frequent guest on your weight-loss lineup.

Or think about this phrase: "Made with Whole Grain." A Harvard study found that just two servings of whole grains a day reduced diabetes risk by 21 percent. But a restaurant can say its bread is "made with whole grain" if there's just a little bit of the stuff sprinkled in there. (That's what you get from Panera Bread's

Whole Grain Baguette—the first ingredient is enriched white flour. You think you're making a strike against diabetes, but you're not!)

What about peanut butter? A study in the *British Journal of Nutrition* found that eating peanut butter during the day helps control blood sugar. But you're eating something more than just peanut butter if you're spooning Jif Natural Peanut Butter Spread onto your toast. The term "spread" indicates it's only about 90 percent real peanut butter, and the rest of it is sugar, palm oil, and molasses.

If that all sounds a bit complicated . . . well, it is. Which is why I've done all the work for you. Instead of just ringing the alarm bells and squawking about troubled foods, I've selected thousands of the healthiest foods in the universe—from America's most popular restaurants, supermarkets, and brands—and broken down just why they're good for you.

I'm not talking about rice cakes here. I'm going to show you how to eat all your favorite foods—and I mean bread and dairy, burgers and fries, ice cream and cookies—and still cut thousands of calories from your diet, all the while cutting your risk of obesity, diabetes, heart disease, depression, and more.

And it's going to be much easier than you thought.

YOUR SIMPLE AND EFFECTIVE HEALTHY EATING GUIDE

To help you navigate the nutritional Narnia, I've created a series of markers that run throughout *Eat It to Beat It!,* a sort of Guided Trail through the American food forest. Throughout this book, I'll be explaining how foods you might think of as indulgences— snacking on Ghirardelli chocolate, for example, or ordering a sirloin steak at TGI Friday's, or adding a little cheese to your

Jack in the Box burger—can actually play an important role in bringing you back to your ideal weight and helping you live a better, longer, happier life.

Here are the guideposts to look for:

 Lose Weight

 Beat Diabetes

 Lower Cholesterol

 Lower Blood Pressure

 Boost Immunity

 Improve Mood

In each case, I'll explain the scientific evidence that demonstrates how eating beef, chocolate, pasta, mayo, even ice cream can boost your health in a number of ways—if you make the right choices, select the right brands, and eat them in the right amounts. Where you see no health-related icon—just a sad, gray tab—the food in question does not by itself harbor a health benefit. But that doesn't mean you have to avoid the food altogether. I'll show you how to avoid the common mistakes that can undermine your health.

From now on, you're never going to have to puzzle out what to order or what to buy. I've done the research for you, comparing tens of thousands of popular restaurant and grocery items, and checking each category to cut down your exposure to unnecessary sugar and calories, unhealthy fats and salt, bizarre flavorings and petroleum-based additives, and ridiculous health claims that serve only to mislead and confuse us. With this simple guide, you'll learn how to:

EAT IT TO BEAT IT! . . . Belly Fat!

I love pasta, how about you? That's why it's great to know that making a simple swap at Olive Garden can change the way you look and feel. If you usually have 5 Cheese Ziti al Forno, try their Linguini Pomodoro (and ask for the whole wheat pasta option). You'll save 680 calories with this swap alone. If you are a regular, make this switch just twice a week and you could *drop 20 pounds this year alone*! Or let's say you wanted to swing by Dairy Queen for a sundae after dinner. A Large Caramel Sundae is a real splurge at 610 calories (get the small and cut that number in half). But it's still a much better choice than their Georgia Mud Fudge Blizzard—a large will cost you 1,490 calories. If you swapped out a big indulgence for a small one like that twice a week, you could cut out nearly 100,000 calories in a year. *That's more than 25 pounds!*

EAT IT TO BEAT IT! . . . High Blood Pressure!

If you've been told to watch your salt intake, then you'd better really come to understand what's in your food. Anyone with a family history of high blood pressure should try to keep their daily sodium intake to no more than 1,500 milligrams a day.

Sounds like plenty, right? But if you're a fan of P.F. Chang's, you might be putting yourself in a less than optimal situation: Their Hot & Sour Soup Bowl contains 7,980 milligrams of sodium, or more than five days' worth. Order their Egg Drop Soup and *save 7,390 milligrams of sodium—and start cutting your risk!*

EAT IT TO BEAT IT! . . . Diabetes!

While you're probably aware that sucking on sugar cubes isn't such a great idea, you'd probably be shocked to discover how often you're getting a huge helping of sugar when you're trying to be healthy. For example, let's say you take the kids to Baskin-Robbins, and those shakes sure look good. But you've heard that the American Diabetes Association has linked sugary drinks to increased risk, so instead of indulging in ice cream, you look for something healthy . . . .like the Mango Banana Smoothie. Well, just one of these "healthy" smoothies is 48 ½ teaspoons of sugar—about five times what you should be consuming in a single day! Treat yourself instead to a cup of Chocolate Chip Cookie Dough: Even the large will save you 162 grams of sugar and 580 calories. That really adds up! Cutting out that many calories twice a week could lead you to drop *nearly 16 pounds in a year*.

EAT IT TO BEAT IT! . . . Colds & Flu!

One recent study found that consuming fish rich in DHA, an omega-3 fatty acid, improves the activity of white blood cells and helps decrease inflammation, giving your immune system a boost. But not all fish are created equal. A piece of broiled Alaskan Chinhook salmon will deliver 1,570 milligrams of omega-3s. A tilapia filet, on the other hand, will give you just 156 milligrams, while also delivering a high dose of unhealthy fats like omega-6s and, if it's fried in the wrong kind of oil, trans fats as well.

EAT IT TO BEAT IT! . . . Brain Fog!

Which came first: Dumb food, or dumb people? Scientists have recently discovered those with the highest intake of trans fatty acids have lower cognitive ability and measurably smaller brains than those with the least. Yet a serving of Pop Secret Buttered Popcorn has nearly three days' worth of trans fat alone. (Talk about "mindless eating"!) You could indulge in Orville Redenbacher's Movie Theater Butter Popcorn and *eliminate brain-shrinking trans fats entirely!*

EAT IT TO BEAT IT! . . . Cholesterol!

Adding just 5 to 10 grams of fiber a day has been shown to lower your cholesterol levels. Does that mean gnawing on drywall? No, how about eating a cookie? You'll get 8 grams of fiber from just two Kashi Oatmeal Dark Chocolate Soft-Baked Cookies, and it will cost you a modest 260 calories. That's right, you could *lower your cholesterol risk—by eating a cookie!*

The restaurant menus have been studied, the nutrition labels analyzed, and the latest research checked and collated. On the following pages, you're going to discover the simplest, easiest health-and-weight-loss guide ever created.

I hope you're hungry!

THE MOST POLLUTED FOODS IN AMERICA

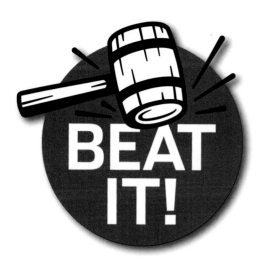

I'm tired of food marketers treating our bellies like landfills. From brain-draining fats to belly-busting sugars, here are the saltiest, saddest, dumbest foods you can eat—and some simple ways to fight back.

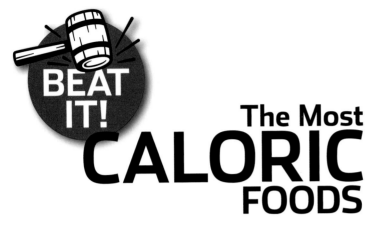

BEAT IT!

The Most CALORIC FOODS

At its most basic, weight gain is about eating more calories than you burn off. So having some idea of how many calories you're eating is probably the most important bit of health information you can have.

Which is why I was stunned to read this on the Cheesecake Factory web page: "At this time, we do not provide nutritional information for our menu selections on our website. We pride ourselves on using only the freshest and finest ingredients available."

Really? I pride myself on having some vague idea of what I put in my mouth on a daily basis. And when you understand just how loaded with unnecessary calories the entrees at Cheesecake Factory are, you can understand why they're trying to play it close to the vest. Luckily some savvy citizens in Washington State (where nutrition labeling is mandatory) scanned the Cheesecake Factory Nutrition Book and made it available online so we were able to see the crazy numbers on their menu. Five of the 10 most caloric foods in America are from one restaurant: Cheesecake Factory.

10 CHEESECAKE FACTORY
Farfalle with Chicken and Roasted Garlic
2,193 calories

9 CHEESECAKE FACTORY
Chicken and Biscuits
2,262 calories

8 UNO CHICAGO GRILL
Super Chi-Town Tasting Plate
2,270 calories

7 CHEESECAKE FACTORY
Pasta Carbonara with Chicken
2,291 calories

6 CHEESECAKE FACTORY
Bistro Shrimp Pasta
2,285 calories

5 CHEESECAKE FACTORY
Beef Ribs
2,306 calories

4 APPLEBEE'S
Appetizer Sampler
2,370 calories

3 TGI FRIDAY'S
Jack Daniel's Ribs and Shrimp with side of parmesan steak fries
2,390 calories

2 FRIENDLY'S
Giant Crowd Pleaser Sundae
2,470 calories

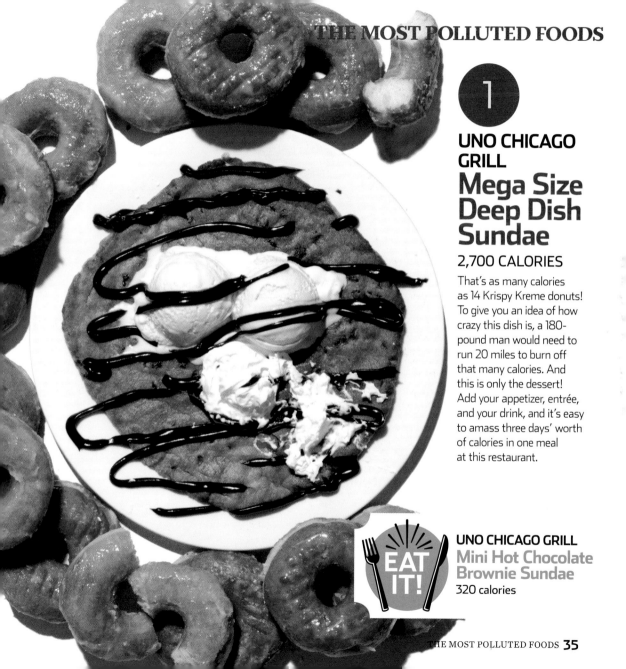

1

UNO CHICAGO GRILL
Mega Size Deep Dish Sundae
2,700 CALORIES

That's as many calories as 14 Krispy Kreme donuts! To give you an idea of how crazy this dish is, a 180-pound man would need to run 20 miles to burn off that many calories. And this is only the dessert! Add your appetizer, entrée, and your drink, and it's easy to amass three days' worth of calories in one meal at this restaurant.

EAT IT!

UNO CHICAGO GRILL
Mini Hot Chocolate Brownie Sundae
320 calories

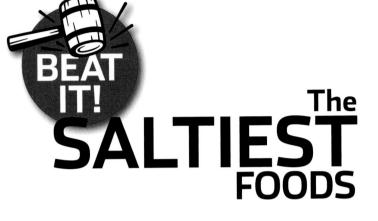

BEAT IT!

The SALTIEST FOODS

Most of us have heard that it's a good idea to "cut down on sodium," but besides making sure the top to the salt shaker is screwed on properly, what does that mean?

Well, first, realize that salt is an essential mineral that your body can't function without. Adults in general should consume no more than 2,400 milligrams (mg) of sodium per day (1,500 if you have high blood pressure, are African American, or are over age 51).

If 2,400 mg sounds like a lot, it is. There's an estimated 189 mg of sodium in one of those little salt packages you get at McDonald's. So if you downed a dozen of them, you'd still be within your daily sodium intake—assuming you didn't eat anything else all day, which you probably wouldn't, because you'd be too busy trying to drain your swimming pool with a flexi-straw.

But a dozen little sodium packages is nothing when you consider what you're getting from these foods, each of which seem saltier than Sarah Silverman's pillow talk.

10 **CHEESECAKE FACTORY**
Sunrise Fiesta Burrito
4,600 mg sodium

9 **CHILI'S**
Boneless Buffalo Chicken Salad
4,720 mg sodium

8 **APPLEBEE'S**
Shrimp Combo Platter
5,200 mg sodium

7 **CHILI'S**
Texas Cheese Fries
5,270 mg sodium

6 **TGI FRIDAY'S**
Jack Daniel's Black Angus Rib-Eye & Grilled Shrimp Scampi*
5,930 mg sodium

5 **ON THE BORDER**
Firecracker Stuffed Jalapeños with Original Queso
6,050 mg sodium

4 **APPLEBEE'S**
Sizzling Skillet Fajitas—Shrimp
6,110 mg sodium

3 **APPLEBEE'S**
Appetizer Sampler
6,120 mg sodium

2 **P.F. CHANG'S**
Dan Dan Noodles
6,190 mg sodium

* (without sides)

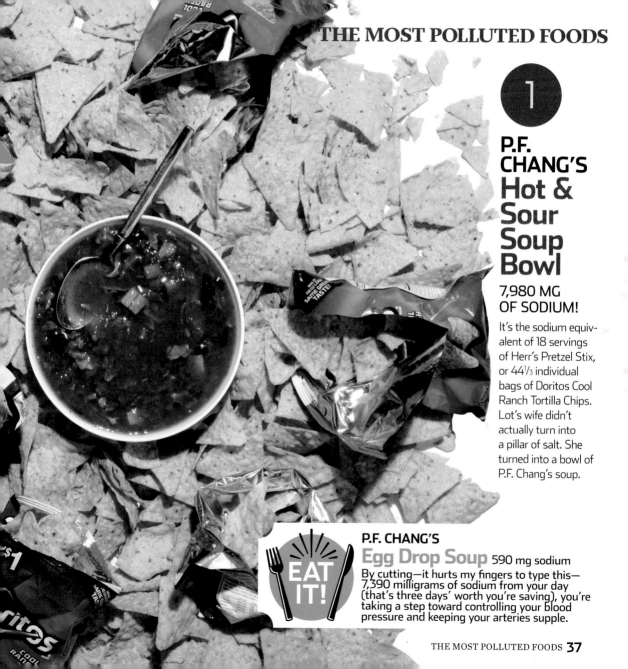

1

P.F. CHANG'S
Hot & Sour Soup Bowl

7,980 MG OF SODIUM!

It's the sodium equivalent of 18 servings of Herr's Pretzel Stix, or 44⅓ individual bags of Doritos Cool Ranch Tortilla Chips. Lot's wife didn't actually turn into a pillar of salt. She turned into a bowl of P.F. Chang's soup.

EAT IT!

P.F. CHANG'S
Egg Drop Soup 590 mg sodium
By cutting—it hurts my fingers to type this—7,390 milligrams of sodium from your day (that's three days' worth you're saving), you're taking a step toward controlling your blood pressure and keeping your arteries supple.

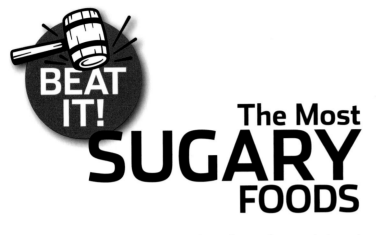

The Most SUGARY FOODS

BEAT IT!

Let's say you're an average American who wants to eat well and live healthfully. And let's say your doctor recommends that to cut your risk of EBS (Enormous Belly Syndrome), you should cut down on added sugar. And The American Heart Association even issued some guidelines:

FOR WOMEN (per day):	FOR MEN (per day):
No more than 25 grams	No more than 38 grams
Which equals: About 6 sugar packets	Which equals: About 9 sugar packets
Or: About 100 calories	Or: About 150 calories

That ought to be easy, right? How hard is it to limit yourself to 6 sugar packets a day?

In a normal world filled with normal food, cutting down on sugar shouldn't be that hard. But in the American food jungle, where nothing is as it appears, added sugar is everywhere. And it's dressed up in funny disguises, like corn syrup and maltodextrin and sucrose.

So beware: Order up some of these overly sweet deals, and you won't be limiting yourself to 6 sugar packets. You'll be lucky to get away with fewer than 60 sugar packets a day!

10 STEAK 'N SHAKE
Chocolate Fudge Brownie Milk Shake—Large
172 grams sugar

9 DUNKIN' DONUTS
Vanilla Bean Coolatta—Large
174 grams sugar

8 STEAK 'N SHAKE
Nutter Butter Milk Shake—Large
184 grams sugar

7 BASKIN-ROBBINS
Bundle of Love Shake
186 grams sugar

6 SONIC
Reese's Peanut Butter Cups Sonic Blast—Large
187 grams sugar

5 DAIRY QUEEN
Lemonade Chiller, Raspberry—Large
189 grams sugar

4 BASKIN-ROBBINS
M&M'S 31º Below Mix-In—Large
190 grams sugar

3 BASKIN-ROBBINS
Mango Banana Smoothie—Large
192 grams sugar

2 CARL'S JR.
Cherry Slushee—(32 oz)
224 grams sugar

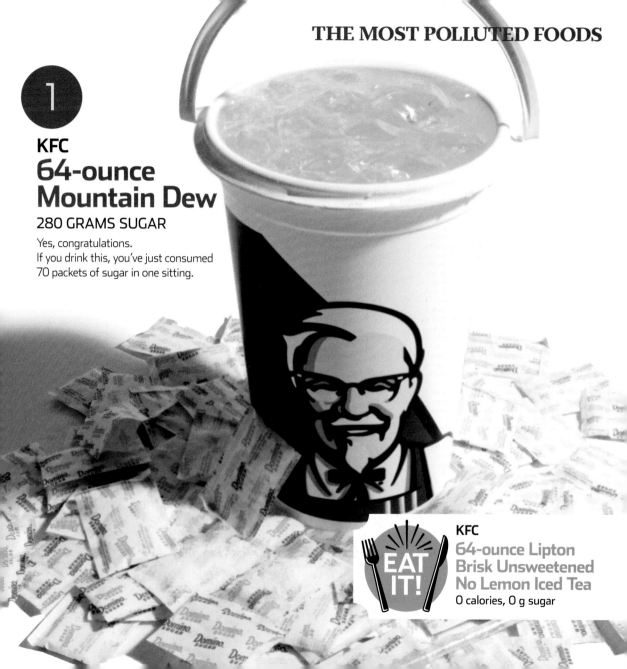

1

KFC
64-ounce Mountain Dew

280 GRAMS SUGAR

Yes, congratulations.
If you drink this, you've just consumed
70 packets of sugar in one sitting.

EAT IT!

KFC
64-ounce Lipton Brisk Unsweetened No Lemon Iced Tea
0 calories, 0 g sugar

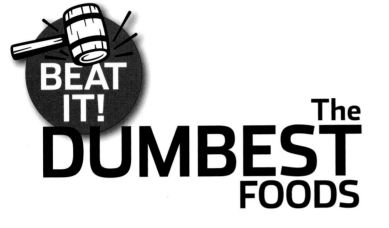

BEAT IT!

The DUMBEST FOODS

Several decades ago, scientists discovered that if they injected vegetable oil with hydrogen, it would turn solid—and stay that way, even at room temperature. Eureka! Suddenly cooking oil became much easier for junk food joints to work with. Unfortunately, these new forms of fat—called trans fats—also caused clogging of the arteries, including those in the brain.

In fact, they impede blood flow so significantly that in studies, those with the most trans fats in their blood have significantly worse cognitive performance—and physically smaller brains!—than those with less trans fats. While trans fats do occur in nature, these natural fats are less dangerous than the artificial kind that go by the moniker "partially hydrogenated oils." In fact, these freaky artificial fats are so bad for you that some municipalities have banned them.

The American Heart Association wants us to get no more than 2 grams of trans fat a day. Yet some food manufacturers seem to think that the dumber we get, the more of their products we'll buy. . . .

10 MARIE CALLENDAR'S
Lattice Apple Pie
3 grams trans fat

9 A&W
Large Fries
4.5 grams trans fat

8 PILLSBURY
Grands Extra Large Easy Split Biscuits
5 grams trans fat

7 POP SECRET
Buttered Popcorn
5 grams trans fat

6 CARL'S JR.
Biscuit 'N' Gravy
7 grams trans fat

5 LONG JOHN SILVER'S
Breaded Clam Strips
7 grams trans fat

4 A&W
Large Breaded Onion Rings
7 grams trans fat

3 LONG JOHN SILVER'S
Battered Onion Rings
7 grams trans fat

2 STEAK 'N SHAKE
Sausage Gravy and Biscuits
8 grams trans fat

LONG JOHN SILVER'S
Baja Fish Taco
9 GRAMS TRANS FAT

Perhaps they should call it the "Bwa-ha-ha" Fish Taco, for the maniacal laughter of the scientists who whipped up a food with nearly five days' worth of trans fats—about as much as you'd find in 18 frozen Banquet Beef Pot Pies. Long John will soon be known as Short Attention Span John if he keeps this up.

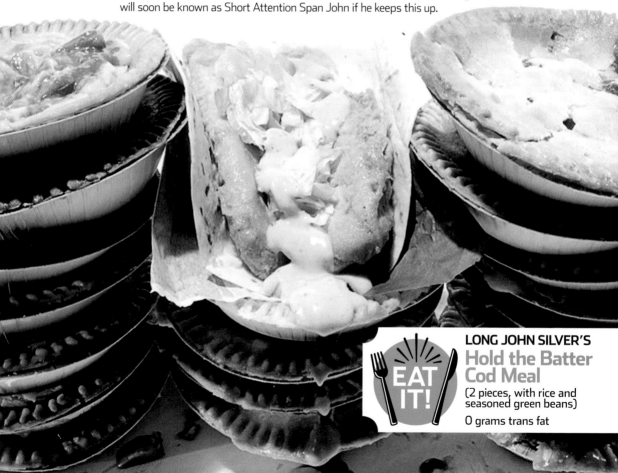

EAT IT!

LONG JOHN SILVER'S
Hold the Batter Cod Meal
(2 pieces, with rice and seasoned green beans)

0 grams trans fat

BEAT IT!

The SADDEST FOODS

Ever feel a little down? There are plenty of pharmaceutical company executives vacationing on private yachts right now, feeling very happy about that.

But here's a secret those executives don't want you to know: Diet has been closely linked to depression, and many of our most popular foods ought to be served with black nail polish and The Cure T-shirts.

Here's why: For good mental and physical health, you need a balance between two fatty acids, omega-3s (from nuts, seeds, fish, and other oily foods) and omega-6s (from cooking oils and grains like corn and soy). In nature they appear in balanced proportions. But processed foods, which come from grains and are often fried in oil derived from grains, are super-high in 6 and often very low in 3. And that's bad: A recent study from the University of South Carolina found that those with the highest intake of omega-6 fatty acids have twice the risk of becoming depressed.

Since depression is closely linked to weight gain and high intakes of omega-6s, it's clear that high-calorie fried foods are the saddest foods in America. Here are the biggest downers, based on their levels of omega-6s.

10 DENNY'S
Fish and Chips
About 60 grams of fat from omega-6

9 ROMANO'S MACARONI GRILL
Parmesan Crusted Sole
About 60 grams omega-6

8 IHOP
Fried Chicken Dinner
About 60 grams omega-6

7 APPLEBEE'S
Chicken Tenders Platter
About 66 grams omega-6

6 RED LOBSTER
Golden Onion Rings
About 75 grams omega-6

5 RED LOBSTER
Crispy Calamari and Vegetables
About 78 grams omega-6

4 APPLEBEE'S
Hand Battered Fish and Chips
About 87 grams omega-6

3 FRIENDLY'S
Kickin' Buffalo Chicken Strips—6 Strips
About 100 grams omega-6

2 APPLEBEE'S
New England Fish & Chips
About 104 grams omega-6

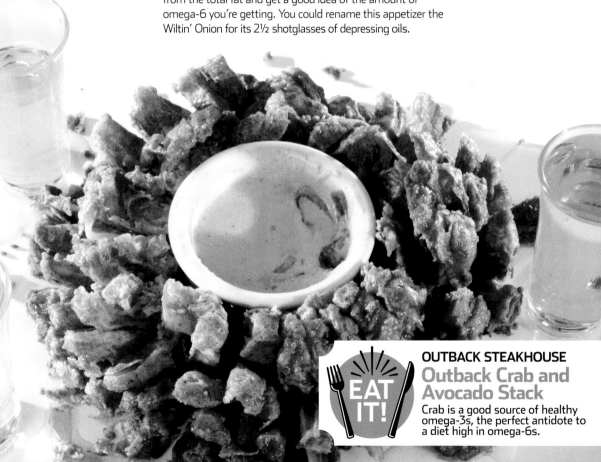

1 OUTBACK STEAKHOUSE
Bloomin' Onion
113 GRAMS OMEGA-6

With deep-fried foods, you can subtract out the saturated fat from the total fat and get a good idea of the amount of omega-6 you're getting. You could rename this appetizer the Wiltin' Onion for its 2½ shotglasses of depressing oils.

EAT IT!

OUTBACK STEAKHOUSE
Outback Crab and Avocado Stack
Crab is a good source of healthy omega-3s, the perfect antidote to a diet high in omega-6s.

BEAT IT!

The FATTIEST FOODS

Fat is good. Fat is delicious. Fat is necessary. And the right kinds of fat—in particular the monounsaturated fats and omega-3 fatty acids you get from certain oils, plants, and fish—is just about the best way to fend off heart disease.

Yet when it comes to bad-for-you saturated and trans fat, today's chain restaurants seem dedicated to slathering it on like an overprotective parent with a bottle of sunscreen. The Centers for Disease Control says that no more than 20 percent to 35 percent of total calories should come from fat. So for a standard 2,000-calorie diet, that means between 44 and 78 grams of fat a day. (A gram of fat is worth 9 calories, for those of you keeping score at home.)

Yet much of what we eat on a regular basis in our favorite chain restaurants carries more than two days' worth of fat—and I'm not talking about the cake and ice cream. What's truly amazing is that of the 10 fattiest foods in America, only one is a dessert—and it barely squeaked onto the list.

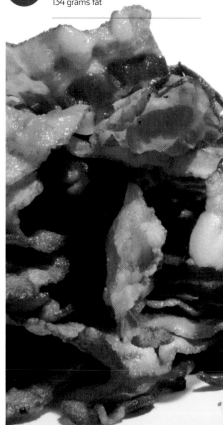

7 ON THE BORDER
Firecracker Stuffed Jalapeños with Original Queso
135 grams fat

6 CHILI'S
Bacon Ranch
Steak Quesadilla
139 grams fat

5 UNO CHICAGO GRILL
Pizza Skins
140 grams fat

4 ON THE BORDER
Border Sampler
142 grams fat

3 UNO CHICAGO GRILL
The Super Chi-Town
Tasting Plate
146 grams fat

2 OUTBACK
STEAKHOUSE
Bloomin' Onion
161 grams fat

1

OUTBACK STEAKHOUSE
Wings
with Medium Sauce

173 GRAMS FAT

That's as much fat as 43 strips of bacon. Outback claims that this offering serves four, but let's be honest: This appetizer is only a dozen wings, which is a typical serving for one at any sports bar; who is going to split it four ways? The Smurfs? Adding arterial insult to injury, you get more than two days' worth of sodium and almost a week's worth of trans fats.

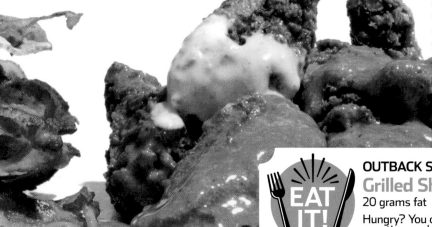

EAT IT!

OUTBACK STEAKHOUSE
Grilled Shrimp on the Barbie
20 grams fat
Hungry? You can get 8 orders of this appetizer and still not reach the fat, calorie, or sodium levels of the wings.

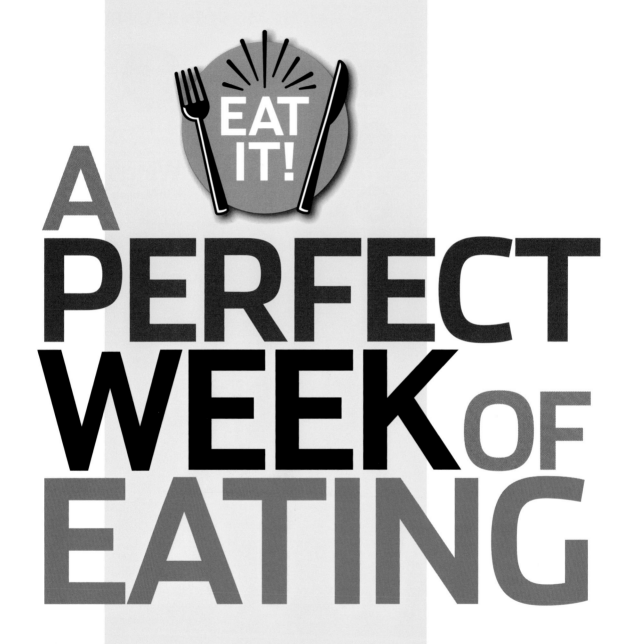

EAT IT!

A PERFECT WEEK OF EATING

This book is filled with smart swaps, enlightening nutritional advice, and weird science facts about food. But what does it all mean, in the end? How can you use *Eat It to Beat It!* to actually change the way you eat, day by day, week by week—and start losing weight and beating back your greatest health risks? And how can you do it without cardboard-like diet food or expensive nutritional supplements or quitting your job to go to culinary school?

Eat It to Beat It! is all about eating your favorite foods—the ones you've been enjoying since childhood—and making smart tweaks (and a handful of easy recipes, when you have time), to strip off the pounds without ever going on a diet. To that end, I've mined through the best products in the supermarket, the top dishes at your favorite restaurants, and some of my own most-loved recipes, and created this never-boring-or-expensive plan for a week of eating for optimum health.

Each day gives you less than 1,700 calories, leaving wriggle room for a snack or two (to maintain a healthy weight, moderately active, adult women should top out at 1,800 calories a day, men at 2,000). But be careful: It's not what you eat that can screw you up, but what you drink. Throw three 16-ounce Mountain Dews into the mix and you've dumped 660 calories of chartreuse sugar on top of your perfectly calculated week.

A PERFECT WEEK OF EATING

	BREAKFAST	LUNCH	DINNER	SNACK
SUNDAY 1,160 total calories	Thin Elvis Oatmeal (page 324) 350 cal	2 Slices Pizza Hut Hand-Tossed Veggie Lovers 360 cal	Halibut a La UPS (page 329) 200 cal	½ cup Häagen-Dazs Vanilla 250 cal
MONDAY 1,610 total calories	The Red, White, & Blue Brain (page 312) 210 cal	Thoughtful Turkey Salad (page 312) 520 cal	Wendy's Jr. Cheeseburger Deluxe with kid's fries 570 cal	Wholly Wholesome Bake at Home Apple Pie 310 cal
TUESDAY 1,060 total calories	Kashi Autumn Wheat Biscuits with ½ cup 1% milk 230 cal	Amy's Organic Lentil Vegetable Soup with 1 slice Vermont Bread Co. Whole Wheat 230 cal	Trouble-Skirting Skirt Steak (page 317) 300 cal	Dairy Queen Small Caramel Sundae 300 cal
WEDNESDAY 1,550 total calories	Starbucks Steel-Cut Oatmeal with Fruit, Nuts & Seeds 220 cal	Helen's Kitchen Fiesta Black-Bean Bowl 290 cal	Longhorn Steakhouse Flo's Filet 880 cal	Cold Stone Creamery Berry Trinity Smoothie 160 cal

	BREAKFAST	LUNCH	DINNER	SNACK
THURSDAY 1,205 total calories	Green Eggs & Ham (page 320) 430 cal	Jack in the Box Grilled Chicken Salad with Low-fat Balsamic Dressing 245 cal	The Bossest Sausage (page 333) 270 cal	2 Kashi Soft Oatmeal Dark Chocolate Cookies 260 cal
FRIDAY 1,261 total calories	Panera Bread Breakfast Power on Whole Grain 340 cal	Kashi Chicken Florentine 290 cal	Carraba Spaghetti Pomodoro on Whole Wheat 431 cal	KIND Fruit and Nut Delight Bar 200 cal
SATURDAY 1,420 total calories	Forgive Us Our Cinnamon Oatmeal (page 332) 450 cal	Subway Roast Beef Sandwich 290 cal	Two to Tango Mango Tacos (page 321) 390 cal	Au Bon Pain Chocolate-Dipped Cranberry Almond Coconut Macaroon 290 cal

EAT IT!

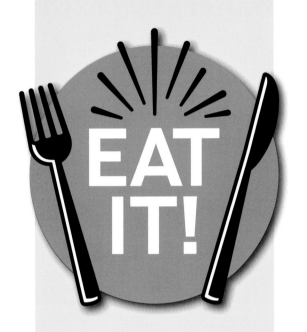

EAT IT!

EAT IT TO BEAT IT!

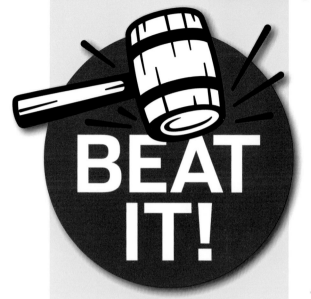

CHAPTER 3

Come with me
on a tour of America's
restaurants and supermarkets
and discover how you can
eat the brands you love—and
start living leaner, healthier,
and happier.

BREAD

Here's what it takes to build a loaf of bread: flour, yeast, salt, sugar, and water. That's it. If you're an evil giant living on top of an enormous beanstalk, maybe you throw in the ground bones of an Englishman. But either way, it's a simple recipe—unless you're cooking for one of the big food companies, in which case you'll also need ingredients like high fructose corn syrup, unsulphured molasses, calcium dioxide, and sorbic acid.

And worse, most commercial breads start with "enriched flour," which is another term for white flour—essentially, wheat that's had the fiber and nutrients yanked out of it. Enriched flour, created by stripping away the nutrition-dense inner and outer layers of the grain, makes bread feel light and fluffy in your mouth, but it turns to sugar pretty much the moment it passes your lips. So what exactly is going into our daily bread? And what's it doing to our bodies?

If there were a section of your supermarket called "Nutrition-Free Zone," this bread would be in it. Not only is it made of mostly enriched flour and high fructose corn syrup, but mixed in with the 27 other ingredients are calcium propionate, an antifungal compound linked to headaches; microcrystalline cellulose (a fiber created by "digesting" wood pulp in hydrochloric acid); and a wee bit of azodicarbonamide, an ingredient also found in yoga mats, rubber gaskets, and the heels of your running shoes.

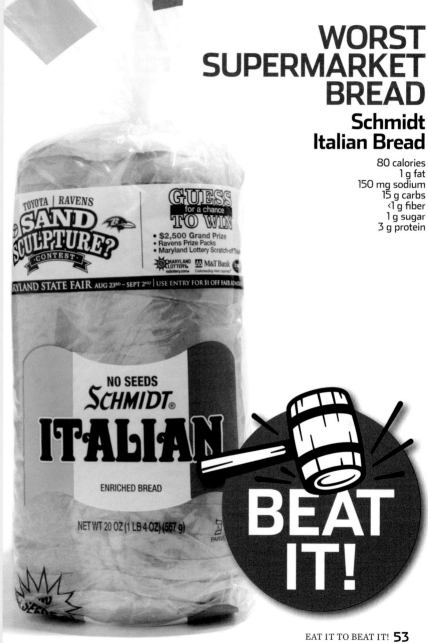

WORST SUPERMARKET BREAD

Schmidt Italian Bread

80 calories
1 g fat
150 mg sodium
15 g carbs
<1 g fiber
1 g sugar
3 g protein

BEAT IT!

How to
EAT IT!
to
BEAT IT!

There are good breads. There are bad breads. There may even be well-meaning but stupid breads. But more and more, there are bad breads being disguised as good breads. "Wheat" breads, "multi-grain" breads, "7/9/12 grain" breads—they all offer the promise of whole-grain goodness, but often the reality is so much less than what's advertised.

THE BREAD RULES

BEWARE WHEAT OR MULTI-GRAIN BREAD. Wait a minute—what? Aren't those good things? Unfortunately, those labels are about as credible as Arnold Schwarzenegger's wedding vows. "Wheat bread" is generally white bread with caramel or molasses added to make it look dark and healthy. "Multi-grain" just means that different kinds of junky refined grains may have been used. Always look for "100% whole wheat" or "100% whole grain" on the package. Or look for the yellow and black whole-grain label, but make sure it says "100% whole grain."

KNOW THE WHOLE STORY. The very first (or second, after water) ingredient should be a whole grain flour: whole wheat, brown rice, whole oats, etc. There shouldn't be any flours listed that don't have the word "whole" next to them.

FIBER UP. Look for breads with at least 2 g of fiber per slice.

DON'T DATEM. DATEM (otherwise known as diacetyl tartaric acid esters of mono- and diglycerides), when mixed with yeast, produces MCPDs (monochloropropanediol isomers), which studies have found to be carcinogenic in animals.

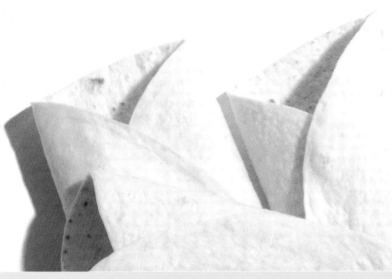

WORST RESTAURANT BREAD
Subway Wrap

310 calories
8 g fat
610 mg sodium
51 g carbs
1 g fiber
8 g protein

Not only is this thin slice of bread 310 calories before you add even the first whiff of meat or sauce, but the ingredient list is a mile long and includes soybean oil and hydrogenated oils as the third and fourth ingredients—which translates to 8 grams of fat per wrap.

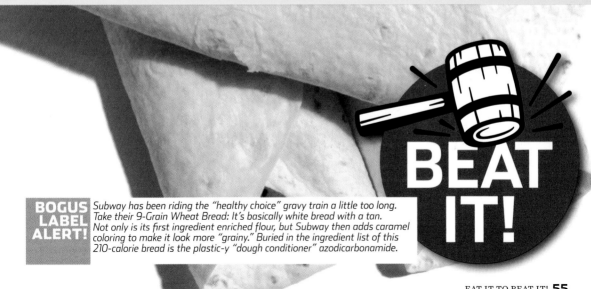

BOGUS LABEL ALERT! *Subway has been riding the "healthy choice" gravy train a little too long. Take their 9-Grain Wheat Bread: It's basically white bread with a tan. Not only is its first ingredient enriched flour, but Subway then adds caramel coloring to make it look more "grainy." Buried in the ingredient list of this 210-calorie bread is the plastic-y "dough conditioner" azodicarbonamide.*

BEAT IT!

EYE THE SIZE. Make sure a serving size is two slices, not one.

AVOID THE YOGA MAT. Azodicarbonamide. Say it with me: azo-di-carbona-mide. You'll find azodicarbonamide in the ingredient lists of some breads, and they call it a bleaching agent or dough conditioner. But it is also used in the production of foamed plastics, the rubber gaskets on glass jars, and synthetic leather (I kid you not), as well as in some pesticides. It has been linked to asthma, which is why products in the UK that contain it must carry a label saying it may cause sensitivities if inhaled.

POP QUIZ!

What's "Bromate?"

1 It's what happens when a "bromance" goes too far.

2 It's something you attach to your broom so it doesn't get jealous of your Swiffer.

That's like experimenting with a drug that Keith Richards refuses to try. . . .

3 It's an ingredient, Potassium Bromate, that's considered by the International Agency for Research on Cancer to be "possibly carcinogenic to humans," and still used in American bread even though it's been banned in Europe, Canada, China, Brazil, and Peru.

Seriously: Should Americans be eating something that even the Chinese have banned?

While the first ingredient in this bread is Unbromated Stone Ground 100% Whole Wheat Flour, the next ingredient is enriched wheat flour, which is basically white flour. So this is by no means "whole grain bread." This bread contains not only high fructose corn syrup, but also something called DATEM (otherwise known as diacetyl tartaric acid esters of mono- and diglycerides). Add in a hefty dose of soy in the form of soy fiber, soy flour, and soybean oil, and you have a bread-like product that still, despite having only 1 g of fiber, somehow carries the American Heart Association HeartCheck label.

WORST "HEALTHY" BREAD
Pepperidge Farm Light Style Bread, Soft Wheat

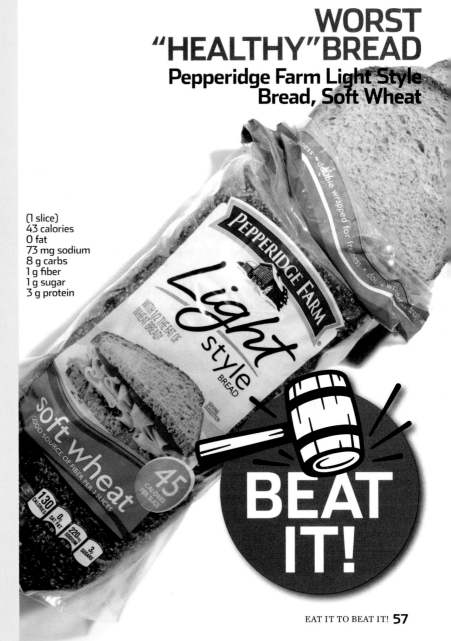

(1 slice)
43 calories
0 fat
73 mg sodium
8 g carbs
1 g fiber
1 g sugar
3 g protein

BEAT IT!

THE WHOLE-GRAIN ADVANTAGE

Boost Immunity

Choose 100 percent whole grains and reap the rewards quickly: A study by the department of food science and technology at the University of Nebraska found that even a short-term intake of whole grains induced compositional alterations of the gut that led to immunological improvements. And a study by the Department of Medicine at the University of Liverpool found that giving subjects selenium, an ingredient in whole grains, allowed them to fend off viruses more effectively.

Lower Blood Pressure

USDA researchers studied 25 adults who replaced refined carbohydrates with whole wheat, brown rice, barley, or half wheat and half barley. After five weeks, systolic blood pressure (the high number you hear at the doctor's office) was reduced by the wheat/rice and combo diet. Diastolic (the low number) was reduced by all four diets, concluding that any whole grains can reduce hypertension and blood pressure.

Lower Cholesterol

The Department of Internal Medicine at Washington University tested cholesterol levels in subjects who ate muffins, some containing whole-wheat germ and some containing refined wheat germ stripped of its naturally occurring nutrients. Those who consumed the whole grains showed a healthier level of cholesterol absorption than those in the refined group.

Beat Diabetes

Whole grains require extensive digestion, while white breads, or those stripped of nutrients, break down at a faster rate, causing a spike in blood glucose levels. Research and studies show that increased intake of whole grains may lower the risk for weight gain, obesity, and as such, type 2 diabetes.

Lose Weight

A 2011 study published by the University of Minnesota School of Public Health shows that whole-grain intake was inversely associated with obesity. And thiamine, a vitamin found in whole grains, was found to impact metabolic function and to also prevent obesity in a Japanese study conducted by the Osaka University of Pharmaceutical Sciences.

Improve Mood

Folate, a vitamin found in whole-wheat bread made without enriched flour, was found to improve treatment outcome in depression.

BOGUS LABEL ALERT! *In 2005, the Whole Grains Council created a Whole Grain Stamp of approval, adding yet another misleading marker to food labels. There are two kinds of Whole Grain Stamps: Basic and 100 percent. Foods with the Basic stamp need only include a little bit of whole grain into their mix. Take Arnold Whole Grain White bread, for example. It carries the basic Whole Grain label, but the first ingredient is unbleached enriched wheat flour. It's as white bread as a Sunday brunch at a Connecticut country club.*

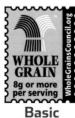

Basic Stamp

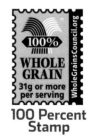

100 Percent Stamp

BEST SUPERMARKET BREAD

Vermont Bread Company
Sodium Free
Whole Wheat

70 calories
1.5 g fat
0 mg sodium
14 g carbs
2 g fiber
<1 g sugar
3 g protein

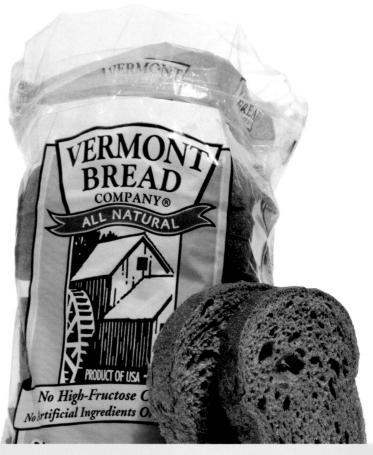

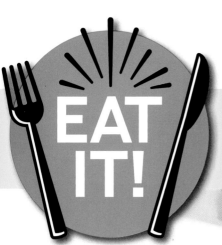

Vermont Bread Company's ingredients are entirely pronounceable. A sandwich made with 2 slices of their Sodium Free Whole Wheat gives you 6 grams of protein and 4 grams of fiber before you even put anything in between.

FOOD FOR LIFE EZEKIEL 4:9 BREAD

Sprouted 100% Whole Grain

80 calories
0.5 g fat
75 mg sodium
15 g carbs
3 g fiber
0 sugar
4 g protein

RUDI'S ORGANIC BAKERY BREAD

100% Whole Wheat

110 calories
1 g fat
150 mg sodium
18 g carbs
3 g fiber
2 g sugar
4 g protein

ALVARADO ST. BAKERY BREAD

Sprouted Whole Wheat

90 calories
0 g fat
180 mg sodium
17 g carbs
2 g fiber
1 g sugar
5 g protein

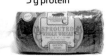

BEST RESTAURANT BREAD

Au Bon Pain's Whole Wheat Multigrain Bread

150 calories
1.75 g fat
30 g carbs
350 mg sodium
5 g fiber
2 g sugar
7 g protein

Restaurant breads, even the "multi-grain" versions, are almost always made with enriched white flour and packed with carbs and salt, but Au Bon Pain offers a relatively healthy, fiber-and-protein-packed whole-grain option.

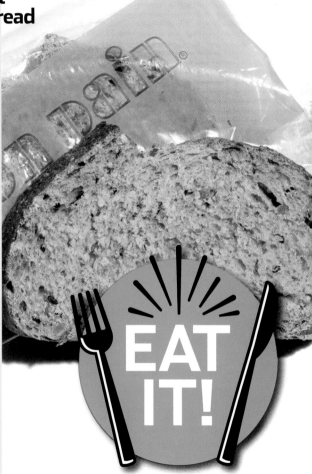

EAT IT!

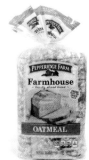

PEPPERIDGE FARM
Farmhouse Bread Oatmeal

120 Calories
1.5 g fat
190 mg sodium
21 g carbs
1 g fiber
3 g sugar
4 g protein

Enriched flour, high fructose corn syrup and sugar, soybean oil, wheat protein isolate

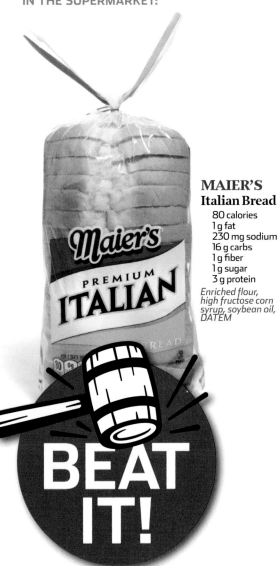

MAIER'S
Italian Bread

80 calories
1 g fat
230 mg sodium
16 g carbs
1 g fiber
1 g sugar
3 g protein

Enriched flour, high fructose corn syrup, soybean oil, DATEM

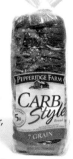

Carb Style Bread 7 Grain

60 calories
1.5 g fat
150 mg sodium
8 g carbs
3 g fiber
0 sugar
5 g protein

First ingredient: 100 percent whole wheat, but also contains wheat protein isolate that contains sulfites, soy fiber, high fructose corn syrup, DATEM, sucralose

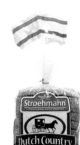

STROEHMANN DUTCH COUNTRY BREAD
100% Whole Wheat

100 Calories
1.5 g fat
200 mg sodium
18 g carbs
3 g fiber
3 g sugar
4 g protein

Another whole-wheat chemistry experiment; high fructose corn syrup, soybean oil, DATEM, azodicarbonamide

BEAT IT!

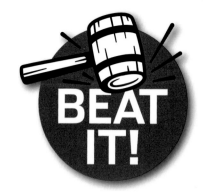

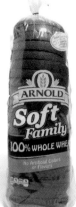

ARNOLD
Soft Family Bread White Whole Grain

140 calories
2 g fat
260 mg sodium
25 g carbs
2 g fiber
4 g sugar
5 g protein

Enriched flour, soybean oil, DATEM, soy lecithin

Whole Grains Health Nut

120 calories
2 g of fat
2 g of fiber

Made with refined flour

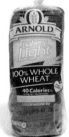

Bakery Light 100% Whole Wheat

40 calories
0.25 g of fat
2.5 g of fiber

Whole wheat, yes, but also made with molasses, monocalcium phosphate, ethoxylated mono- and-diglcerides, azodi- carbonamide

FIBER ONE Country White

100 calories
1 g fat
200 mg sodium
24 g carbs
6 g fiber
4 g sugar
4 g protein

Enriched flour, sugar, sugarcane fiber, honey, high fructose corn syrup (4 sugars), soy bean oil, soy lecithin, DATEM

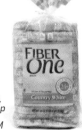

IN RESTAURANTS:

SUBWAY
Italian Bread

Italian bread is white bread. In addition to enriched flour, it contains DATEM and azodicarbonamide

200 calories
2 g fat
270 mg sodium
38 g carbs
1 g fiber
5 g sugar
7 g protein

Quiznos
Artisan Wheat

Contains colorings and sulfites

190 calories
2.5 g fat
35 g carbs
410 mg sodium
2 g fiber
3 g sugar
7 g protein

PANERA
Whole Grain Loaf

It's made primarily with enriched white flour

130 calories
1g fat
27 g carbs
290 mg sodium
3 g fiber
2 g sugar
6 g protein

Whole Grain Baguette

Ditto

140 calories
1g fat
29 g carbs
310 mg sodium
3 g fiber
2 g sugar
6 g protein

BREAKFAST CEREALS

Walking down the cereal aisle of your supermarket is like taking a spin through Taylor Swift's date book: It's filled with an array of colorful, bizarre characters making heady, stirring promises—but most of them just want to break your heart.

And protecting your heart—not to mention your waistline—is hard when there are more than 100 brands of cereal calling out for your attention in your average supermarket. But let's assume that you already know that boxes with charming leprechauns, tricky rabbits, and crunchy captains aren't good for you. If you're buying one of these cartoon characters, you're buying a box that ought to say Breakfast Sugar—with Cereal Added!

Problem is, choosing a healthy breakfast cereal isn't just a matter of eliminating the animated spokescreatures. A lot of healthy-sounding cereals are just as candy-like as the brand that the terrific tiger sells. So that's the bad news.

The good news: If your healthy cereal lets you down, at least you won't have to read about it in the tabloids, and then sit down and write a hit song about it. . . .

This "Special" cereal needs some remedial education. See the big hunk of chocolate on the front of the box? Looks good, but note the term "chocolatey," which is market speak for "does not contain real chocolate." The FDA regulates the use of the word "chocolate" and this cereal contains only chocolate-like ingredients. With a mere 3 grams of fiber and only 2 grams of protein, it contains 62 percent more sugar than fiber and 75 percent more sugar than protein.

WORST "HEALTHY" COLD CEREAL
Kellogg's Special K Chocolatey Strawberry

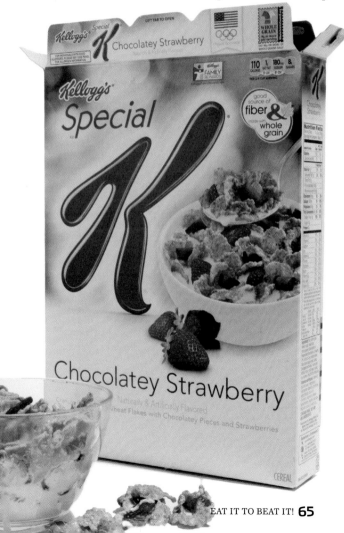

BEAT IT!

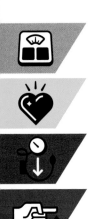

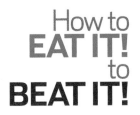

How to
EAT IT!
to
BEAT IT!

In a normal world, cereal in milk would be the best, healthiest way to start your day.

That's because you want to begin your morning with as much nutrition as possible, but with the focus on two important factors: fiber and protein. Both fill you up with slow-burning energy that boosts your fat-burning metabolism and keeps you full and satisfied into the afternoon. A traditional cereal mix of whole grains, maybe with some chopped nuts in there, would give you plenty of fiber, and the nuts and milk would give you a healthy dose of protein. Soooo . . . what went wrong?

THE CEREAL RULES

LOOK OUT FOR IMPOSTERS. Words like "froot" or "choco-latey" are a sure sign that you're not getting what you think you're getting. Most likely these foods don't contain chocolate or fruit, but a mixture of sugars, fats, flavors, and dyes to make it seem like they do.

AVOID "YOGURT-COVERED." Those cereals that claim to have yogurt in them really just have "yogurt powder" mixed with trans-fatty oils and flavorings so that it sticks to whatever they're trying to cover in "yogurt."

STEER CLEAR OF THE THREE C'S: "CRUNCH," CRISPS," AND "CLUSTERS." These words usually mean that there are clumps of crispy rice held together by sugar and fat. Tasty! But more candy-like than breakfast-like. And they don't add any whole grain goodness . . . they subtract.

Here's a phrase for you: "Flavored and Colored Fruit Pieces." That's taken right from Quaker's ingredient list. And what they've done is taken dried apples or figs and injected them with corn syrup solids, corn starch, and partially hydrogenated vegetable oil (trans fat!), mixed in something called a "creaming agent," which is also made of trans fats, and dyed the resulting concoction various fruity colors using things like artificial blueberry color, Blue 2 Lake, and Red 40 Lake. And yet, the nutrition label still says it contains 0 g trans fats.

TIP: If you want blueberries in your oatmeal, then buy some and add them in yourself.

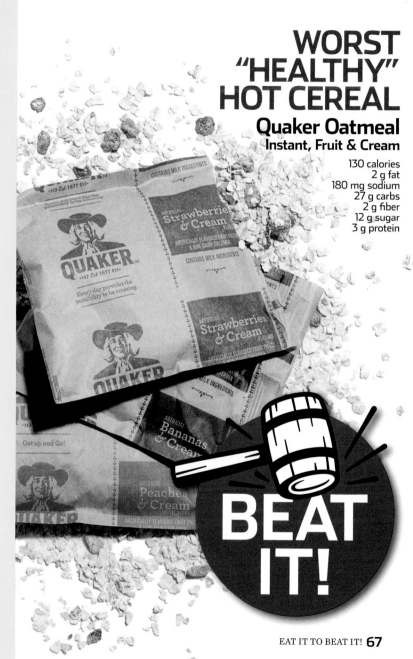

WORST "HEALTHY" HOT CEREAL

Quaker Oatmeal
Instant, Fruit & Cream

130 calories
2 g fat
180 mg sodium
27 g carbs
2 g fiber
12 g sugar
3 g protein

BEAT IT!

FIND REAL WHOLE GRAINS. Manufacturers love to slap claims on the front label about how many grams of whole grains you'll get by choosing their product. But always compare those with the serving size on the nutrition facts label—if the front label shouts 10 g of whole grains per serving, but the serving size is 30 g, that means it's mostly a refined grain cereal, which you want to avoid.

UNDERSTAND THE SUGAR GAME

- Check the Sugar Numbers. The American Heart Association's added sugar threshold is no more than 24 grams of sugar (about 6 teaspoons) for most women and no more than 36 grams of sugar (about 9 teaspoons) for most men. So a reasonable rule for your breakfast cereal is that it should constitute no more than a third of that. So, you're looking for 6 to 8 grams of sugar per serving.
- Now Check the Numbers Again. Compare the number of sugar grams in a serving to the overall number of grams in a serving. Sometimes, a serving of cereal will be as low as 24 grams; if your cereal has 12 grams of sugar in it, then your cereal is basically 50 percent sugar . . . and you're eating candy for breakfast.
- Look for the Synonyms. Sugar comes in a lot of forms, but that's exactly what you're getting if the label has any of the following: evaporated cane juice, barley malt, dextrose, corn syrup, molasses, sucrose, fructose, high-fructose corn syrup, corn syrup solids, brown sugar, or the 50 or so other names sugar hides behind. If sugar or any of its secret identities are within the first two or three items listed in the ingredient list, skip it.

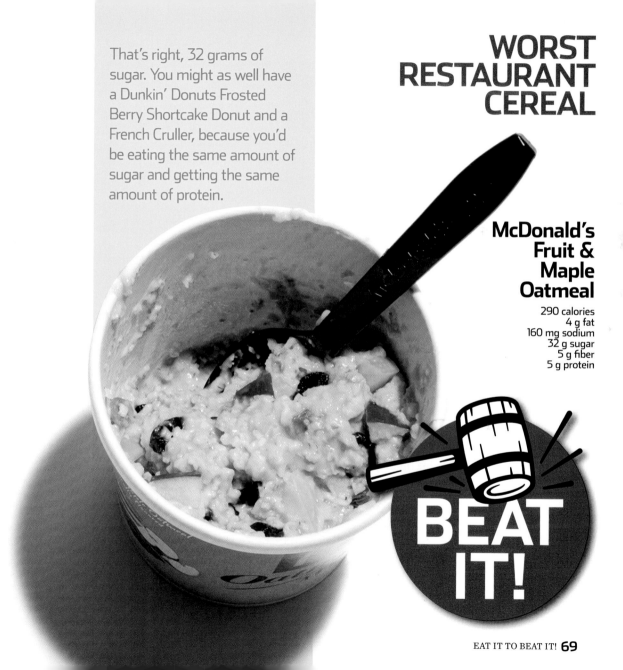

That's right, 32 grams of sugar. You might as well have a Dunkin' Donuts Frosted Berry Shortcake Donut and a French Cruller, because you'd be eating the same amount of sugar and getting the same amount of protein.

WORST RESTAURANT CEREAL

McDonald's Fruit & Maple Oatmeal

290 calories
4 g fat
160 mg sodium
32 g sugar
5 g fiber
5 g protein

BEAT IT!

THE CEREAL ADVANTAGE

Lose Weight

Multiple observational studies have linked whole grain intake and grain fiber to lower body weight and body fat, as well as greater success with weight loss, according to the U.S. Department of Agriculture's Nutrition Evidence Library.

Beat Diabetes

Research has also linked whole grains to a decreased risk for diabetes. A 2007 study from Harvard looked at whole grain, bran, and germ intake using data from the Nurses' Health Studies and found that two servings per day of whole grains reduced diabetes risk by 21 percent. Another study, published in 2013 in the *American Journal of Clinical Nutrition,* found that higher consumption of whole grains also helped stop the progression of insulin resistance that leads to prediabetes.

Lower Cholesterol

Whole grain cereals can be a good source of both soluble and insoluble fiber, and many epidemiological studies have linked a diet high in fiber to significantly lower risk for heart disease as a whole. But when it comes to cholesterol, it seems the type of fiber matters; only soluble fiber works to lower cholesterol. Whole grain oats and oat bran, ingredients in many modern cereals that are rich in soluble fiber, are proven to be helpful for lowering LDL cholesterol. This suggests that to really maximize the cholesterol-lowering effects of whole grains, you might be better off eating oatmeal for breakfast.

Lower Blood Pressure

Male doctors who reported eating whole-grain cereals seven days a week had a 20 percent lower risk for hypertension, according to a study presented at the 2011 American Heart Association conference. A smaller study, published in 2010 in the *American Journal of Clinical Nutrition,* found that increasing intake of whole grains to 3 servings a day, including a whole-grain cereal, decreased blood pressure significantly.

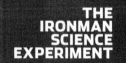

THE IRONMAN SCIENCE EXPERIMENT

Want to portray a billionaire scientific genius like Robert Downey, Jr.? Or just amaze and disgust your friends? Here's something gross to chew on. You know how so many cereals are "fortified with iron"? What that often means is that powdered iron filings are added to the flours used to make the cereals. And unlike iron that occurs naturally in plants and other foods, these filings are not very well absorbed and used by our bodies—we just pass most of them through, and never actually get the benefits of said iron. Here's a little experiment you can do at home so you can see for yourself just what you've been eating all these years.

Find a cereal that contains fortified iron in the ingredient list, like Special K, Corn Flakes, Life, or Kellogg's All-Bran Complete Wheat Flakes.

Pour the cereal into a bowl and crush it until it's a fine powder (a mortar and pestle work great for this part).

Pour the powdery cereal onto a piece of white paper and run a strong magnet right over the top of the pile (refrigerator magnets probably aren't strong enough).

Check out the little bits of black iron on the end of your magnet. Good morning!

BEST RESTAURANT CEREAL

220 calories
5.5 g fat
0 mg sodium
5 g fiber
5 g sugar
7 g protein

Starbucks Steel-Cut Oatmeal

with Old-Fashioned Rolled Oats, with Fruit, Nut & Seed Medley topping

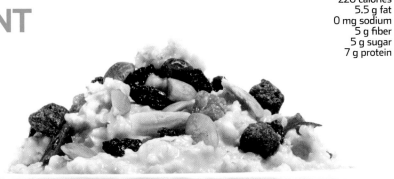

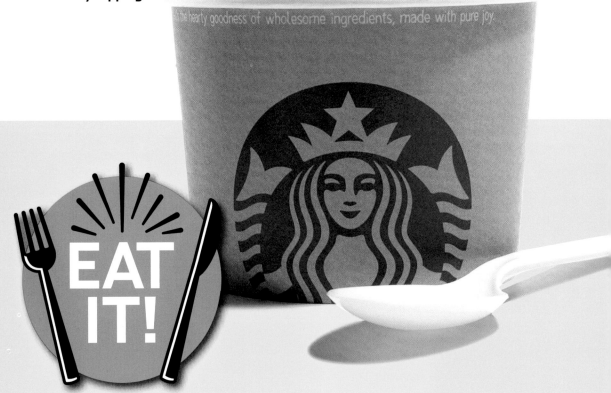

the hearty goodness of wholesome ingredients, made with pure joy.

EAT IT!

COSI
Oatmeal
- 149 calories
- 47 mg sodium
- 4 g fiber
- 1 g sugar
- 5 g protein

DENNY'S
Grits with butter
- 220 calories
- 3 g fat
- 15 mg sodium
- 3 g fiber
- 0 g sugar
- 5 g protein

BURGER KING
Quaker Oatmeal Original
- 140 calories
- 3.5 g fat
- 100 mg sodium
- 3 g fiber
- 1 g sugar
- 5 g protein

The two main girders of a smart breakfast —protein and fiber— become really convenient when you can snag both with your morning latte. Load it up with fruit and nuts—not sugar or syrup—and Starbucks' oatmeal becomes the easy solution to a busy morning.

DENNY'S
Oatmeal with milk and brown sugar
- 240 calories
- 5 g fat
- 220 mg sodium
- 3 g fiber
- 27 g sugar
- 6 g protein

FRIENDLY'S
Raisin Bran Crunch
- 370 calories
- 3 g fat
- 390 mg sodium
- 6 g fiber
- 40 g sugar
- 11 g protein

Perhaps the most unfriendly cereal around, this really unfortunate breakfast is just an oversized serving of Kellogg's original cereal. But if you finish your bowl, you'll get as much sugar as 3½ bowls of Froot Loops!

IHOP
Simple & Fit Super Fruit Oatmeal
- 290 calories
- 3.5 g fat
- 15 mg sodium
- 7 g fiber
- 29 g sugar
- 6 g protein

JAMBA JUICE
Steel Cut Blueberry & Blackberry Oatmeal
- 290 calories
- 3.5 g fat
- 25 mg sodium
- 6 g fiber
- 25 g sugar
- 8 g protein

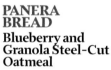

PANERA BREAD
Blueberry and Granola Steel-Cut Oatmeal
- 320 calories
- 9 g fat
- 160 mg sodium
- 8 g fiber
- 21 g sugar
- 6 g protein

BURGER KING
Quaker Oatmeal Maple Brown Sugar Flavor
- 270 calories
- 4 g fat
- 290 mg sodium
- 5 g fiber
- 29 g sugar
- 5 g protein

BEST COLD CEREALS

Kashi
Autumn Wheat
Whole Wheat
Biscuits

180 calories
1 g fat
0 sodium
6 g fiber
7 g sugar
6 g protein

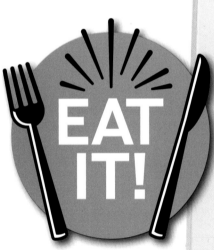

EAT IT!

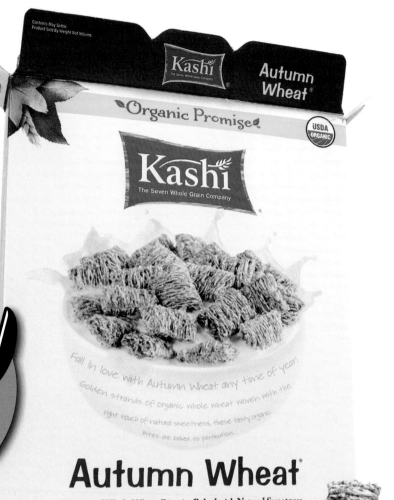

Made from three ingredients starting with organic whole-grain wheat, this cereal provides 50 grams of whole grains and 0 salt, and only 7 grams of sugar. It's also Non-GMO Project Verified and doesn't taste like cardboard.

BARBARA'S CEREAL
Shredded Wheat

140 calories
1 g fat
0 mg sodium
5 g fiber
0 mg sugar
4 g protein

KELLOGG'S
All Bran

80 calories
1 g fat
80 mg sodium
10 g fiber
6 g sugar
4 g protein

UNCLE SAM CEREAL

190 calories
5 g fat
135 mg sodium
10 g fiber
1 g sugar
7 g protein

MULTIGRAIN CHEERIOS

110 calories
1 g fat
120 mg sodium
3 g fiber
6 g sugar
2 g protein

WHEAT CHEX

160 calories
1 g fat
270 mg sc
6 g fiber
5 g sugar
5 g proteir

HONEY BUNCHES OF OATS
Greek Honey Crunch

230 calories
3.5 g fat
160 mg sodium
4 g fiber
13 g sugar
5 g protein

Contains "Greek Yogurt Style Coating" which is basically palm kernel oil, sweetener, and heat-treated yogurt powder. Translation: not yogurt.

BASIC 4

200 calories
2 g fat
280 mg sodium
4 g fiber
13 g sugar
4 g protein

Sugar is in the ingredient list 6 times, not to mention artificial color and flavor

---

QUAKER
Oh's

110 calories
2 g fat
170 mg sodium
1 g fiber
12 g sugar
1 g protein

Artificial flavors, 5 different sugars

KELLOGG'S
Raisin Bran Crunch

190 calories
1 g fat
200 mg sodium
4 g fiber
19 g sugar
4 g protein

6 different sugars in the ingredient list, plus artificial flavors

Cracklin' Oat Bran Cereal

200 calories
7 g fat
135 mg sodium
6 g fiber
14 g sugar
4 g protein

Artificial flavors, high sugar, and palm oil, which is high in saturated fat

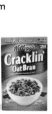

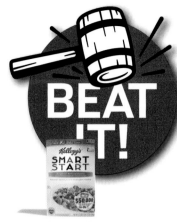

BEAT IT!

Smart Start Cereal Original Antioxidants

190 calories
1 g fat
210 mg sodium
3 g fiber
14 g sugar
4 g protein

6 different sugars in the ingredient list, plus artificial flavors and colors

KASHI
Go Lean Crunch

190 calories
3 g fat
100 mg sodium
8 g fiber
13 g sugar
9 g protein

High sugar, with 16 g of whole grain, this is only 30 percent whole-grain cereal

BEST
HOT CEREAL
Quaker Oat Bran

150 calories
3 g fat
0 mg sodium
6 g fiber
1 g sugar
7 g protein

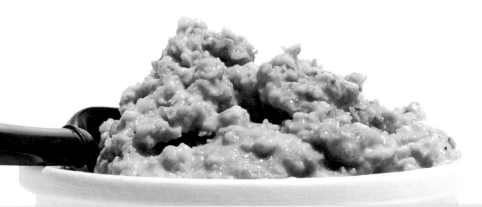

One ingredient: Oat Bran. It also packs 6 grams of fiber and 7 grams of protein.

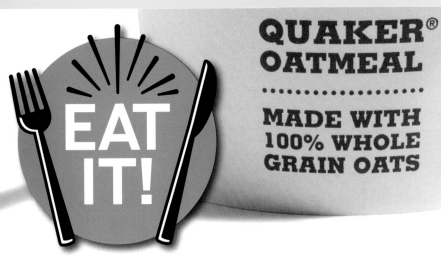

EAT IT!

QUAKER® OATMEAL

MADE WITH 100% WHOLE GRAIN OATS

QUAKER OATS
Old Fashioned
- 150 calories
- 3 g fat
- 0 mg sodium
- 4 g fiber
- 1 g sugar
- 5 g protein

OLD WESSEX LTD.
Irish Style Oatmeal
- 150 calories
- 3 g fat
- 0 mg sodium
- 4 g fiber
- 0 g sugar
- 6 g protein

BOB'S RED MILL
Old Fashioned Organic Rolled Oats
- 160 calories
- 2.5 g fat
- 0 mg sodium
- 4 g fiber
- 1 g sugar
- 7 g protein

McCANN'S
Irish Oatmeal Quick Cooking
- 150 calories
- 2 g fat
- 0 mg sodium
- 4 g fiber
- 0 g sugar
- 4 g protein

HODGSON MILL
Hot Cereal Oat Bran All Natural
- 120 calories
- 3 g fat
- 0 mg sodium
- 6 g fiber
- 0 g sugar
- 6 g protein

QUAKER
Real Medleys Oatmeal+ Summer Berry
- 250 calories
- 3 g fat
- 250 mg sodium
- 7 g fiber
- 14 g sugar
- 8 g protein

A little high in sugar, but uses real fruit, which is the source of some of that sugar, and has few ingredients

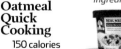

QUAKER
Instant Oatmeal Maple & Brown Sugar Lower Sugar
- 120 calories
- 2 g fat
- 290 mg sodium
- 3 g fiber
- 4 g sugar
- 4 g protein

Artificial flavors, caramel color, which has been linked to cancer, and sucralose, an artificial sweetener linked to inflammation and cellular damage

Instant Oatmeal Dinosaur Eggs Maple & Brown Sugar
- 190 calories
- 3.5 g fat
- 260 mg sodium
- 3 g fiber
- 14 g sugar
- 4 g protein

Trans fat in the form of partially hydrogenated oils, even though it says 0 g trans fat, artificial colors, artificial flavors, caramel coloring

Weight Control Oatmeal, Instant Maple & Brown Sugar
- 160 calories
- 3 g fat
- 290 mg sodium
- 6 g fiber
- 1 g sugar
- 7 g protein

Artificial flavors, caramel color, and sucralose

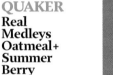

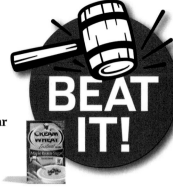

BEAT IT!

INSTANT CREAM OF WHEAT
Hot Cereal Maple Brown Sugar
- 130 calories
- 0 g fat
- 140 mg sodium
- 1 g fiber
- 13 g sugar
- 2 g protein

High in sugar and caramel color

KASHI
Heart to Heart Instant Oatmeal Golden Maple
- 160 calories
- 2 g fat
- 260 mg sodium
- 5 g fiber
- 12 g sugar
- 4 g protein

High sugar for something claiming to be heart healthy

BURGERS

In the latter years of a long-ago millennium—I'm talking about the late '80s—everything was bigger than it is today. Hair was bigger. Shoulder pads were bigger. Cell phones were bigger. Eddie Murphy's career was bigger. Today's postmillennial society is practically Dinklagesque compared to the oversized swagger of the Reagan years.

But in that long-ago era of amplitude, one thing was a lot smaller: our hamburgers. The average hamburger once stood at a reasonable 333 calories. Nowadays, it's hard to find a sit-down restaurant that serves a burger less than three times that size. What's behind these bulbous, bulging burgers? Let's investigate.

BOGUS LABEL ALERT! *"100 Percent Beef." "Certified Angus." "No additives or fillers." Sounds like you're getting nothing but ground cuts of meaty cow, right? But burgers carrying these labels can still be partially comprised of "lean finely textured beef," otherwise known as pink slime—mechanically separated bits of skeletal muscle, skin and bone fragments that are then treated with ammonium hydroxide as an antimicrobial intervention. A 3.2-ounce beef patty containing 15 percent LFTB will contain up to 40 mg of ammonia. The folks at Certified Angus Beef say that it may be present at low levels (less than 10 percent) in some of their ground chuck.*

Order a burger at Ruby Tuesday, and prepare for Regret Wednesday. Every burger there tops 1,200 calories, even their turkey burger. But the pretzel burgers deserve their own circle of hell: Consider that Jake's Wayback offers a Triple Triple Burger with 9 patties and 9 slices of cheese, and holds a contest every year challenging people to down one of these monstrosities. Yet Jake's creation has only 140 more calories and a third less sodium than Ruby's "everyday" entree!

WORST RESTAURANT BURGER

Ruby Tuesday Bacon Cheese Pretzel Burger

1,759 calories
105 g fat
3,257 mg sodium
9 g fiber
68 g protein

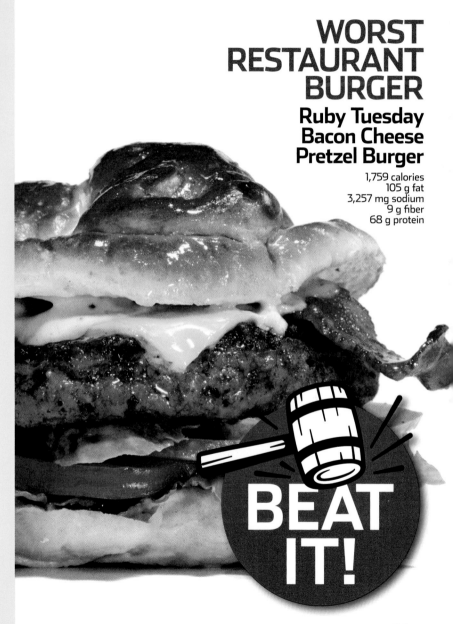

BEAT IT!

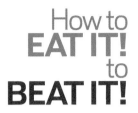

How to
EAT IT!
to
BEAT IT!

Too often, what you're getting when you bite into a burger is a big mouthful of something more like Hamburger Helper. Except there's nothing helpful about ground bone, E. coli, soy protein, and anything else that isn't straight-up moo cow.

THE BURGER RULES

THINK PINK SLIME. Look for the words "Contains no finely textured beef" on the label, or pick out a nice cut of chuck, sirloin, or round and have the butcher at the supermarket grind it for you (they do this!). Also, "Certified Angus" ground round and ground sirloin don't contain pink slime.

DON'T JUDGE BEEF BY ITS COLOR. Supermarket beef is usually treated with carbon monoxide to keep its red color. The only way to tell if beef has gone bad is to smell it.

GO FOR THE GRASS. To avoid getting up close and personal with superbugs, consider buying meat that's labeled "organic" or "grass-fed." (NOTE: The only national chain restaurants serving grass-fed or organic beef are Chipotle, Moe's Southwest Grille, and Elevation Burger. Or go to eatwell.com and search for grass-fed beef at restaurants near you.)

DON'T BUY BOGUS LABELS. Labels claiming "No Antibiotic Residues," "Antibiotic Free," or "No Antibiotic Growth Promotants" aren't actually verified by the USDA. You're only clear of antibiotics if the meat carries the red, white, and blue USDA Process Verified shield.

The folks at Certified Angus Beef say that "lean finely textured beef" (LFTB) may be present in some of their ground chuck, which is what Bubba Burger Certified Angus Beef Chuck burgers are made from. Another term for LFTB: pink slime.

430 calories
35 g fat
90 mg sodium
0 fiber
0 sugar
26 g protein

WORST SUPERMARKET BURGER

Bubba Burger Certified Angus Beef Chuck burgers

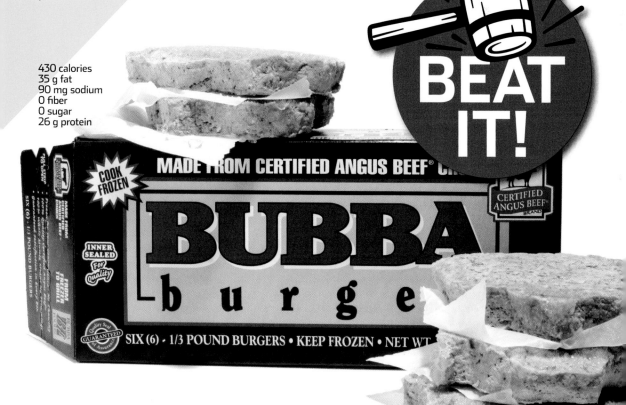

BEST RESTAURANT BURGER

Wendy's Jr. Cheeseburger Deluxe

350 calories
19 g fat
830 mg sodium
2 g fiber
7 g sugar
17 g protein

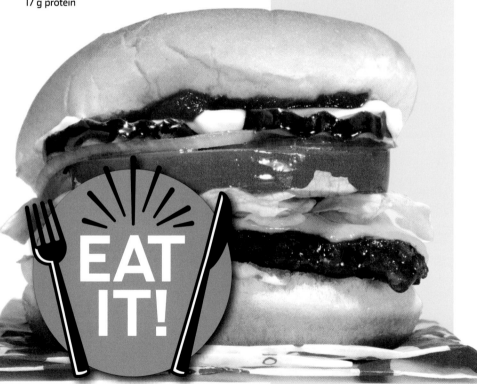

EAT IT!

Swapping out a Dave's Hot & Juicy with Cheese (see opposite page) for a Jr. Cheeseburger Deluxe will save you 770 calories and more than 1,000 mg of sodium, the latter of which will be good for your blood pressure!

STEAK'N SHAKE
Single Steakburger with cheese

330 calories
16 g fat
570 mg sodium
<1 g fiber
5 g sugar
15 g protein

MCDONALD'S
Grilled Onion Cheddar

310 calories
13 g fat
66 mg sodium
2 g fiber
7 g sugar
15 g protein

BURGER KING
Cheeseburger

280 calories
12 g fat
690 mg sodium
1 g fiber
7 g sugar
15 g protein

ELEVATION BURGER
Elevation Burger
(double meat wrapped in lettuce)

370 calories
24 g fat
390 mg sodium
1 g fiber
1 g sugar
41 g protein

IN-N-OUT BURGER
Cheeseburger with onion
(mustard and ketchup instead of spread)

400 calories
18 g fat
1,080 mg sodium
3 g fiber
10 g sugar
22 g protein

CARL'S JR.
The Super Bacon Six Dollar Burger

- 1,040 calories
- 66 g fat
- 2 g trans fat
- 2,230 mg sodium
- 3 g fiber
- 10 g sugar
- 56 g protein

WENDY'S
Dave's Hot 'n Juicy ¾ lb Triple with Cheese

- 1,120 calories
- 69 g fat
- 1,990 mg sodium
- 3 g fiber
- 11 g sugar
- 69 g protein

HARDEE'S
⅔ lb Monster Thickburger

- 1,300 calories
- 93 g fat
- 2,860 mg sodium
- 3 g fiber
- 5 g sugar
- 59 g protein

BURGER KING
Triple Whopper

- 1,020 calories
- 65 g fat
- 1,090 mg sodium
- 3 g fiber
- 13 g sugar
- 58 g protein

APPLEBEE'S
Quesadilla Burger
(without fries)

- 1,400 calories
- 105 g fat
- 3.5 g trans fat
- 3,260 mg sodium
- 6 g fiber
- 72 g protein

CHILI'S
Southern Smokehouse Burger

- 1,600 calories
- 96 g fat
- 4,490 mg sodium
- 8 g fiber
- 18 g sugar
- 65 g protein

TGI FRIDAY'S
Jack Daniel's Burger

- 1,360 calories
- 73 g fat
- 3,500 mg sodium
- 6 g fiber
- 49 g protein

FRIENDLY'S
Grilled Cheese Burger

- 1,540 calories
- 92 g fat
- 2,490 mg sodium
- 9 g fiber
- 10 g sugar
- 55 g protein

RED ROBIN
Whiskey River BBQ Burger

- 1,408 calories
- 89 g fat
- 1,717 mg sodium
- 6 g fiber
- 47 g protein
- 21 g sugar
- 47 g protein

IN THE SUPERMARKET:

BALL PARK
Beef Patty Flame Grilled Fully Cooked

- 230 calories
- 19 g fat
- 440 mg sodium
- 0 g fiber
- 0 g sugar
- 15 g protein

Contains partially hydrogenated soybean oil (trans fats), corn syrup, and some kind of "beef," which doesn't inspire confidence

The Applebee's Quesadilla Burger: Double the calories of their hamburger

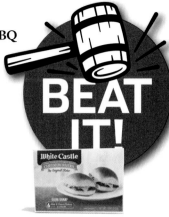

WHITE CASTLE
Cheeseburgers

- 310 calories
- 17 g fat
- 600 mg sodium
- 1 g fiber
- 3 g sugar
- 14 g protein

Their ingredient list just says "beef," and their burger buns have a bit of azodicarbonamide (plastic foam used in yoga mats)

BANQUET BURGER
Sliders

- 280 calories
- 14 g fat
- 5 g sat fat
- 510 mg sodium
- 2 g fiber
- 3 g sugar
- 12 g protein

Beef (no idea what grade) is mixed with textured soy protein and water

CAKES & BAKED DESSERTS

There's a reason cake is the go-to dessert for birthday parties, retirement sendoffs, and strippers who need something to jump out of. Unlike its frequent companion, ice cream, cake doesn't have even the slightest claim to any health benefits; it's really just a candy sponge with candy icing on top.

That said, there's a difference between the devil you know and the devil's food cake you don't. The best bad-for-you desserts are just what they appear to be. But others have ingredients that take bad and turn it into cruel and unusual.

1,679 calories
49 g sat fat
970 mg sodium
206 g carbs

WORST RESTAURANT DESSERT

Cheesecake Factory Chocolate Tower Truffle Cake

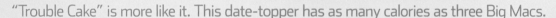

"Trouble Cake" is more like it. This date-topper has as many calories as three Big Macs.

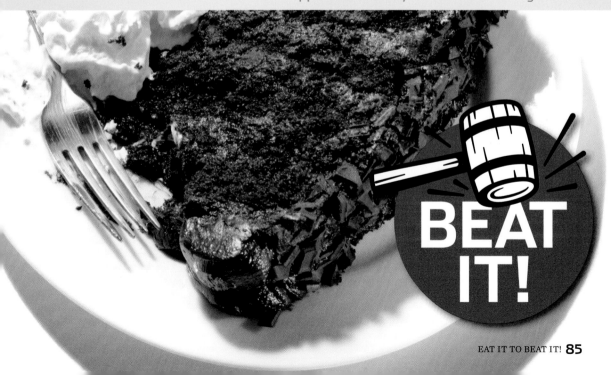

BEAT IT!

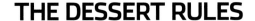

THE DESSERT RULES

WATCH FOR TRANS FATS. They're just as likely to secretly lurk in ingredient lists as they are to boldly show their face on nutrition panels. If you see "partially hydrogenated oil" of any kind, keep moving.

KEEP IT CLEAN. The fewer ingredients, the better. Flour, sugar, eggs, and butter taste amazing together. Why ruin a good thing with extra fillers, gums, fats, and flavors?

DON'T INDULGE ALONE. Eating dessert as part of a family ritual will make the cake taste even better, according to research published in the journal *Psychological Science*. Rituals allow us to savor food more.

NUTRITION QUIZ

Which of the following is "partially hydrogenated"?

A totally incompetent competitor at a hot air balloon race	Your 2-year-old nephew after an epic Pampers fail	A transgender patient who runs out of money at the worst possible time

None of the above. "Partial hydrogenation" refers to the process of forcibly bonding hydrogen atoms to liquid fats like vegetable oil to make them into solids. In food uses, this process results in the creation of trans fats, which are considered so toxic to your circulatory system that some municipalities have banned them from restaurant use altogether. ("Fully hydrogenated" oils don't have trans fats.) The American Heart Association recommends you have no more than 2 grams of trans fats a day, but less is better. The problem: By law, a food with less than 0.5 grams of trans fat can still say "0 g trans fat." So you need to read the ingredient list.

Trans fatty acids are not found in nature, but they are found in our food, and Marie Callender's pie takes the cake. One serving has three times as much trans fat as the American Heart Association wants you to eat in a whole day.

WORST SUPERMARKET DESSERT

Marie Callender's Small Apple Pie

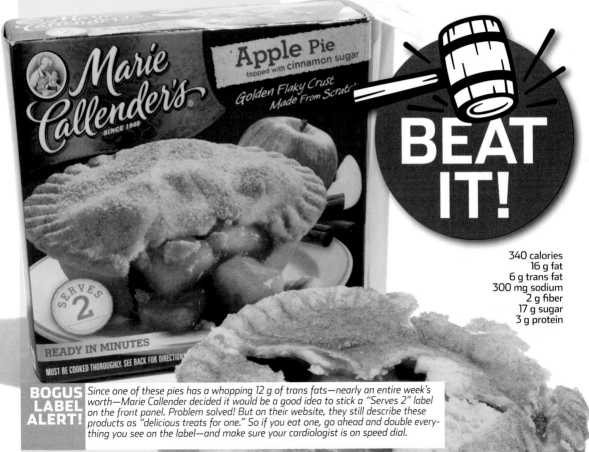

BEAT IT!

340 calories
16 g fat
6 g trans fat
300 mg sodium
2 g fiber
17 g sugar
3 g protein

BOGUS LABEL ALERT! *Since one of these pies has a whopping 12 g of trans fats—nearly an entire week's worth—Marie Callender decided it would be a good idea to stick a "Serves 2" label on the front panel. Problem solved! But on their website, they still describe these products as "delicious treats for one." So if you eat one, go ahead and double everything you see on the label—and make sure your cardiologist is on speed dial.*

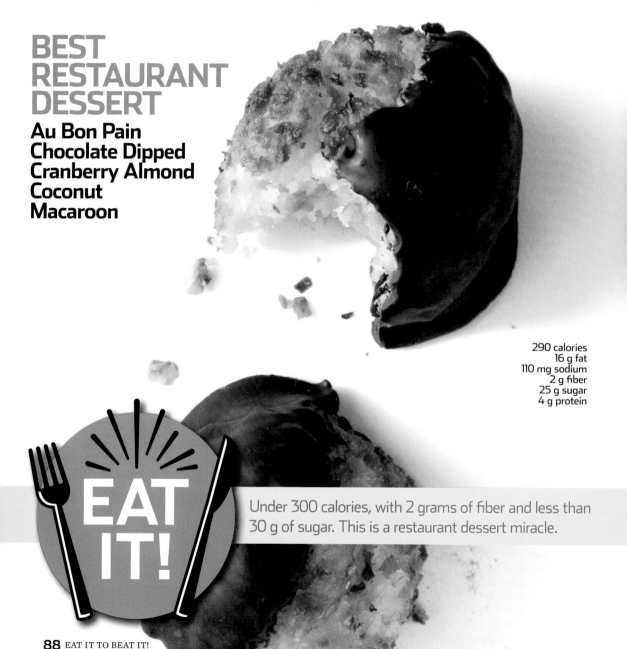

BEST RESTAURANT DESSERT

**Au Bon Pain
Chocolate Dipped
Cranberry Almond
Coconut
Macaroon**

290 calories
16 g fat
110 mg sodium
2 g fiber
25 g sugar
4 g protein

EAT IT!

Under 300 calories, with 2 grams of fiber and less than 30 g of sugar. This is a restaurant dessert miracle.

P.F. CHANG'S
Tiramisu
- 250 calories
- 15 g fat
- 60 mg sodium
- 1 g fiber
- 4 g protein

LONG JOHN SILVER'S
Chocolate Cream Pie
- 280 calories
- 17 g fat
- 230 mg sodium
- 1 g fiber
- 19 g sugar
- 3 g protein

BLIMPIE
Brownie
- 230 calories
- 10 g fat
- 115 mg sodium
- 1 g fiber
- 21 g sugar
- 3 g protein

HARDEE'S
Peach Cobbler (small)
- 285 calories
- 7 g fat
- 230 mg sodium
- 1 g fiber
- 45 g sugar
- 1 g protein

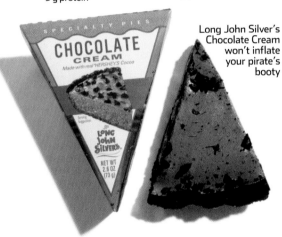

Long John Silver's Chocolate Cream won't inflate your pirate's booty

CARL'S JR.
Chocolate Cake
- 300 calories
- 12 g fat
- 350 mg sodium
- 1 g fiber
- 36 g sugar
- 3 g protein

KFC
Cafe Valley Bakery Lemon Cake
- 210 calories
- 11 g fat
- 190 mg sodium
- 0 g fiber
- 19 g sugar
- 2 g protein

TGI FRIDAY'S
Tennessee Whiskey Cake
- 1,270 calories
- 54 g fat
- 820 mg sodium
- 5 g fiber
- 15 g protein

CHILI'S
Skillet Chocolate Chip Cookie
- 1,430 calories
- 71 g fat
- 930 mg sodium
- 6 g fiber
- 115 g sugar
- 16 g protein

P.F. CHANG'S
The Great Wall of Chocolate
- 1,520 calories
- 72 g fat
- 1,400 mg sodium
- 10 g fiber
- 18 g protein

The Applebee's Blue Ribbon Brownie: like eating 5½ cream pies

OUTBACK STEAKHOUSE
Chocolate Thunder From Down Under
- 1,554 calories
- 105 g fat
- 562 mg sodium
- 6 g fiber
- 122 g sugar
- 20 g protein

FRIENDLY'S
Caramel Fudge Oreo Brownie Sundae
- 1,410 calories
- 66 g fat
- 620 mg sodium
- 2 g fiber
- 124 g sugar
- 19 g protein

APPLEBEE'S
Blue Ribbon Brownie
- 1,600 calories
- 77 g fat
- 910 mg sodium
- 7 g fiber
- 20 g protein

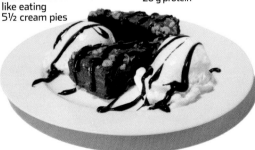

BEAT IT!

BEST SUPERMARKET DESSERT

Vitalicious VitaBrownie Deep & Velvety Chocolate

100 calories
2 g fat
105 mg sodium
10 g fiber
10 g sugar
4 g protein

No trans fats, made with real ingredients, and loaded with fiber, light on the sugar. . . . You won't find a healthier dessert option on the shelves.

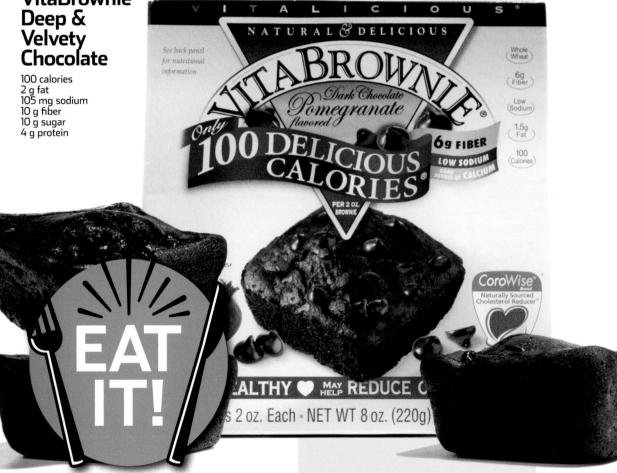

See back panel for nutritional information.

VITALICIOUS®

NATURAL & DELICIOUS

VITABROWNIE®
Dark Chocolate
Pomegranate
flavored

Only 100 DELICIOUS CALORIES®

PER 2 OZ. BROWNIE

6g FIBER
LOW SODIUM
GOOD SOURCE OF CALCIUM

Whole Wheat
6g Fiber
Low Sodium
1.5g Fat
100 Calories

CoroWise™ Brand
Naturally Sourced
Cholesterol Reducer™

...EALTHY ♥ MAY HELP REDUCE C...

...s 2 oz. Each • NET WT 8 oz. (220g)

EAT IT!

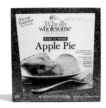

WHOLLY WHOLESOME

Bake At Home Pie, Apple

310 calories
14 g fat
40 mg sodium
3 g fiber
27 g sugar
3 g protein

GILLIANS

Fruit Pie, 9 Inch, Pumpkin

350 calories
15 g fat
350 mg sodium
3 g fiber
22 g sugar
5 g protein

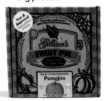

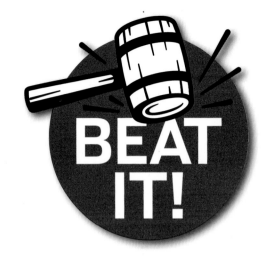

BEAT IT!

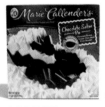

MARIE CALLENDER'S

Chocolate Satin Pie Frozen Thaw & Serve

580 calories
38 g fat
4 g trans fat
330 mg sodium
3 g fiber
33 g sugar
5 g protein

⅙th of a cake

PEPPERIDGE FARM

3-Layer Cake Coconut Frozen

240 calories
10 g fat
1.5 g trans fat
120 mg sodium
<1 g fiber
25 g sugar
1 g protein

⅛th of a cake

Besides trans fats, this cake also includes propylene glycol. You know it as antifreeze

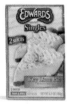

EDWARDS PIE

Singles Key Lime

330 calories
16 g fat
0 g trans fat
240 mg sodium
42 g sugar
6 g protein

⅛th of a cake

While it might say 0 trans fat, partially hydrogenated vegetable oil is on the ingredients list, along with hydroxypropyl methylcellulose, a lubricant for contact lenses

CHEESE

The word "cheese" has two meanings:

- a dairy product that's cultured

- a tacky, synthetic item that's totally lacking in culture

More and more, when you buy something that you think is #1, you're actually getting something more like #2—a once "natural" food product that's become as plastic as a $5 Kmart hairpiece.

Consider, if you will, your typical slice of American cheese. In most cases, you're buying something called "pasteurized processed cheese food"—which means you're getting a product that needs to be only 51 percent cheese. The rest of it could be salt, butter, soy, preservatives, and any number of strange additives. And the key phrase is "cheese food," because sometimes your cheese slice will be something called a "cheese product"—they don't even dare call it food—which means you're eating something that's less than 51 percent cheese.

Confused yet? Don't worry, I'll set you straight. . . .

BOGUS LABEL ALERT!

If one of the ingredients in your cheese were ground wood chips digested in sodium hydroxide, would you consider it "organic"? The earnest folks who work at Horizon Organic do. On the label of their finely shredded cheddar cheese is the word "cellulose," which means processed wood chips. It's categorized as a synthetic ingredient, but the FDA, apparently pining for the timber industry, allows its use in foods labeled "natural" and "organic." Horizon people: It's bad enough that you're calling it "organic;" at least tell us what your product really is: Shredded Cheese & Trees!

SHREDDED:

Kraft 2% Milk Shredded Mozzarella

70 calories
5 g fat
1 g carbs
180 mg sodium
0 fiber
0 sugar
7 g protein

Not only does this low-fat cheese have 180 mg of salt per serving, you're also getting a nice helping of wood pulp to go with it.

SOLID:

Heluva Good Natural Cheese, Reduced Sodium Cheddar

This low-sodium cheese uses potassium chloride to make up for the lack of salt. It's considered safe by the FDA; however, people with kidney or heart problems should avoid it. And isn't heart and kidney health the reason you're avoiding salt in the first place?

110 calories
9 g fat
25 mg sodium
0 fiber
0 sugar
7 g protein

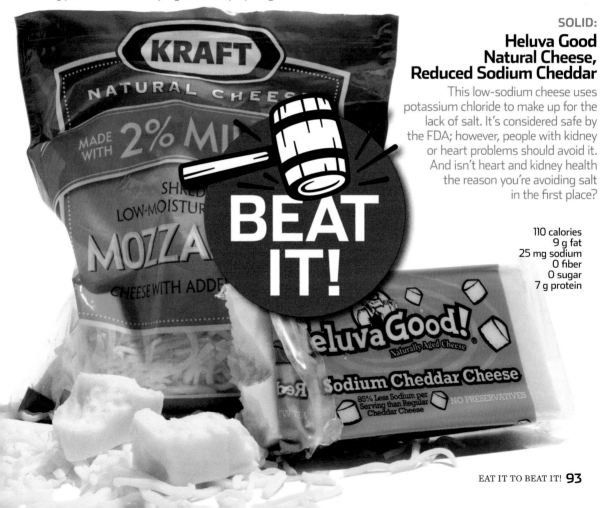

BEAT IT!

How to EAT IT! to BEAT IT!

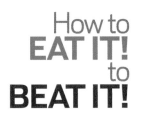

Is regular, full-fat cheese evil? And is it really better to eat low-fat, processed stuff with the soy and the butter and the shredded trees and the potassium chloride (yes, the stuff they use in lethal injections)?

Bottom line: No. Although low-fat dairy is still the recommendation of the Dietary Guidelines for Americans, the American Heart Association, and the American Diabetes Association, the research is beginning to suggest otherwise. For example, a 2013 study published in the *European Journal of Nutrition* found that people who ate more high-fat dairy products had no higher risk for heart or metabolic diseases, and on top of that, they actually had a lower risk for obesity.

According to a recent article in *The Nutrition Source,* published by the Harvard School of Public Health, in the 1960s, fats and oils supplied Americans with about 45 percent of calories, and about 13 percent of adults were obese; less than 1 percent had type 2 diabetes, a serious weight-related condition. Today, Americans take in less fat, getting about 33 percent of calories from fats and oils. Yet nowadays 34 percent of adults are obese and 11 percent have diabetes, most with type 2 diabetes. If fat and saturated fat were really the problem, wouldn't these numbers be completely different? Evidence is mounting that the culprit isn't fat; it's all the stuff they put in there to make food "low-fat." Here's what you need to know before you, um, cut the cheese.

THE CHEESE RULES

KEEP IT SIMPLE. You don't need much more than milk, salt, and enzymes to make good cheese. Full-fat cheese will have fewer weird things in it.

READ THE SMALL PRINT. The FDA mandates that processed cheeses be labeled according to the percentages of actual cheese in the product (see the handy chart at right).

SHRED YOUR OWN. I know it's easy to open a bag and pull out shredded cheese, but if you're reading this book, you must be a little concerned about what's in your food. You don't need to be eating wood pulp, which is added to shredded cheese to keep it from sticking together.

BONUS: GO GRASS FED. This isn't always an option, but dairy from grass-fed cows has a fatty acid profile that is extremely healthy. Grass-fed dairy has fewer calories and more antioxidants, and while there is naturally less fat in grass-fed dairy, that fat that is in there contains more omega-3s, including 5 times more conjugated linoleic acid, a healthy fat that has been shown to protect against cancer, heart disease, and obesity.

THE REAL CHEESE ADVANTAGE

Before you select something low-fat and cheese-like, consider what benefits you'll get if you buy the real deal.

♥ Lower Cholesterol

A study published in a 2012 issue of the *American Journal of Clinical Nutrition* found that a higher intake of saturated fat from dairy was associated with a lower risk for heart disease. But in comparison, higher intakes of saturated fat from meat raised risk for heart disease, leading the researchers to conclude that it may be the source of saturated fat that matters.

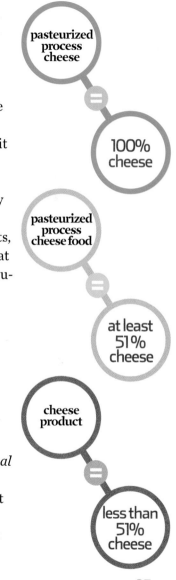

pasteurized process cheese

= 100% cheese

pasteurized process cheese food

= at least 51% cheese

cheese product

= less than 51% cheese

Lose Weight

A study of close to 2,000 Swedish men published in the *Scandinavian Journal of Primary Health Care* found that those who ate more dairy fat actually had less belly fat.

Another study in the *European Journal of Clinical Nutrition* documented a modest increase in the appetite-controlling hormone PYY in people who ate full-fat dairy, suggesting that cheese could be a useful tool for controlling hunger and food cravings.

Boost Immunity

A study from 2010 in the journal *FEMS Immunology & Medical Microbiology* found that cheese may help stop age-related deterioration of immune response thanks to qualities that make it a great carrier of probiotic or "good" bacteria. Elderly people given a daily piece of probiotic gouda experienced a clear increase of circulating natural killer cells and other immune markers. But it seems that most manufacturers haven't taken advantage of this as there are few probiotic cheeses on the market.

THE CHEESIEST (AND UNCHEESIEST) RESTAURANTS

It's hard enough to understand what's in your cheese when you're buying it yourself in the supermarket. But when it's on a burger or a grilled cheese from your local restaurant? Nearly impossible. Here's what we were able to detect.

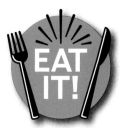

PANERA BREAD

Classic Grilled Cheese

They use organic American cheese that contains no soy, just milk, salt, enzymes, and a little sodium citrate (a harmless derivative of citric acid)

JACK IN THE BOX

You can order your burgers with real cheddar cheese instead of processed American

ELEVATION BURGER

They use real cheddar cheese and offer blue cheese too

CHIPOTLE MEXICAN GRILLE

Real Monterey Jack cheese and real cheddar cheese, grated in the restaurant, no wood pulp!

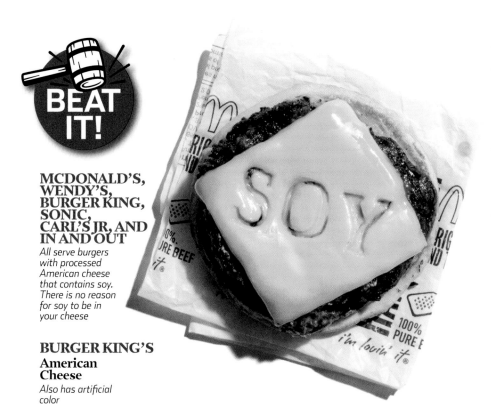

MCDONALD'S, WENDY'S, BURGER KING, SONIC, CARL'S JR, AND IN AND OUT

All serve burgers with processed American cheese that contains soy. There is no reason for soy to be in your cheese

BURGER KING'S

American Cheese

Also has artificial color

BEST CHEESE

BEST CREAM CHEESE:

Breakstone's Temp Tee Whipped Cream Cheese

80 calories
8 g fat
5 g sat fat
65 mg sodium
1 g protein

Only 80 calories and barely any sodium for this real cream cheese.

BEST AMERICAN SINGLES:

Horizon Organic American Singles

60 calories
5 g fat
3 g sat fat
230 mg sodium
3 g protein

Why make a grilled cheese with creepy processed stuff, when Horizon's product is made from nothing but organic milk products, salts, and enzymes.

BEST COTTAGE CHEESE:

Daisy 4% Cottage Cheese

110 calories
5 g fat
3g sat fat
360 mg sodium
13 g protein

High in sodium, like most cottage cheeses, but a whopping 13 g of protein for just 110 calories, and nothing but dairy and salt in the ingredient list.

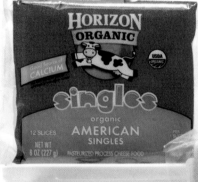
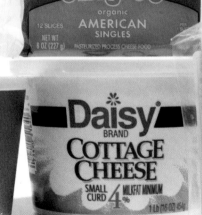
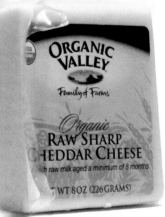

EAT IT!

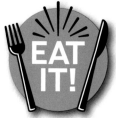

BEST BLOCK CHEESE:

Organic Valley Grassmilk Raw Sharp Cheddar

110 calories
9g fat
6 g sat fat
170 mg sodium
7 g protein

Higher in omega-3 fatty acids, CLA (another heart-healthy fat), and calcium than cheese from grain-fed cows, this is as healthy as you can get.

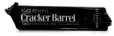

CRACKER BARREL
Aged Reserve Extra Sharp Cheddar

120 calories
10 g fat
6 g sat fat
180 mg sodium
6 g protein

KERRYGOLD
Vintage Dubliner Irish Cheese

110 calories
9 g fat
5 g sat fat
200 mg sodium
7 g protein

CABOT
Vermont Cheese Premium Naturally Aged Cheddar Seriously Sharp

110 calories
9 g fat
6 g sat fat
180 mg sodium
7 g protein

LOCATELLI
Pecorino Romano

110 calories
9 g fat
6 g sat fat
480 mg sodium
7 g protein

SUN-NI
Armenian String Cheese

80 calories
6 g fat
3.5 g sat fat
220 mg sodium
7 g protein

WEIGHT WATCHERS
String Cheese Light Low-Moisture Part-Skim Mozzarella

50 calories
2.5 g fat
1 g sat fat
150 mg sodium
6 g protein

ORGANIC VALLEY
Neufchatel Cheese Organic

80 calories
6 g fat
4 g sat fat
115 mg sodium
2 g protein

FRIENDSHIP
Cottage Cheese

90 calories
2.5 g fat
6 g sat fat
360 mg sodium
14 g protein

APPLEGATE
Natural American Cheese

80 calories
7 g fat
5 g sat fat
270 mg sodium
5 g protein

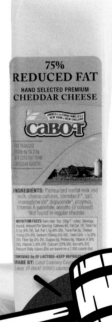

75% REDUCED FAT
HAND SELECTED PREMIUM
CHEDDAR CHEESE

CHEDDAR:
CABOT
Vermont Cheese, Sharp Cheddar, 75% Reduced Fat

60 calories
2.5 g fat
1.5 g sat fat
200 mg sodium
9 g protein

This cheese might have a few less grams of fat in it, but they replaced it with more salt and added cornstarch and mono- and diglycerides to hold the cheese together.

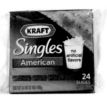

AMERICAN SINGLES:
KRAFT
American Singles

60 calories
4 g fat
2.5 g sat fat
200 mg sodium
0 g fiber
3 g protein

The Kraft American Single is not technically a cheese but a "pasteurized prepared cheese product," which means it's at best only 50 percent cheese. You'll find cheesier singles on Craig's List. . . .

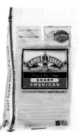

LAND O' LAKES
Yellow American Cheese

100 calories
9 g fat
5 g sat fat
400 mg sodium
5 g protein

One slice gives you one-fifth of your daily sodium intake. And who eats just one slice?

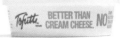

CREAM CHEESE:
TOFUTTI
Better Than Cream Cheese

60 calories
5 g fat
1.5 g sat fat
120 mg sodium
1 g protein

This product says "no butterfat," "no cholesterol," and "Better Than Cream Cheese" right on the side in large letters. However, its main ingredient after water is partially hydrogenated soybean oil, which is a trans fat—the most unhealthy kind of fat there is!

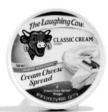

LAUGHING COW
Smooth Sensations Cream Cheese Spread

45 calories
4 g fat
2.5 g sat fat
140 mg sodium
2 g protein

Is the cow laughing, or burping due to the carrageenan used in this product, which can cause abdominal inflammation?

BEAT IT!

COTTAGE CHEESE:

BREAKSTONE'S LIVEACTIVE
2% Cottage Cheese
90 calories
2 g fat
1.5 g sat fat
380 mg sodium
10 g protein

BOGUS LABEL ALERT!

While this LIVEACTIVE cottage cheese is made from cultured milk, it also contains inulin, a prebiotic that is supposed to feed the good bacteria that's already in your gut, but some studies suggest that it feeds the bad bacteria, too.

FIBER ONE
Cottage Cheese, Lowfat, with Fiber
80 calories
2 g fat
1.5 g sat fat
430 mg sodium
10 g protein

More sodium and less protein than you should be getting . . . must mean something weird's in there (in this case, the very non-cheesey polysorbate 80)

SHREDDED CHEESE:

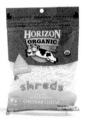

HORIZON ORGANIC
Cheddar Cheese, Finely Shredded
110 calories
9 g fat
5 g sat fat
180 mg sodium
7 g protein

We still don't like eating wood chips

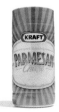

KRAFT CHEESE
Parmesan, 100% Grated
20 calories
1.5 g fat
75 mg sodium
2 g protein

More wood chips

Here's what you're getting from 1 ounce of your favorite cheese

CURDS OF WISDOM

CHEESE TYPE	CALORIES	FAT g	SAT FAT g	PROTEIN	SODIUM mg
FETA	75	6.03	4.237	4.03	260
CAMEMBERT	85	6.88	4.326	5.61	239
WHOLE MILK MOZZARELLA	85	6.34	3.729	6.29	178
PASTEURIZED AMERICAN	94	7.27	4.269	4.78	364
BRIE	95	7.85	4.936	5.88	178
CREAM CHEESE	97	9.71	5.469	1.68	103
BLUE	100	8.15	5.293	6.07	323
PROVOLONE	100	7.55	4.842	7.25	248
EDAM	101	7.88	4.982	7.08	230
GOUDA	101	7.78	4.994	7.07	232
MUENSTER	104	8.52	5.419	6.64	178
COTTAGE CHEESE	104	0.42	0.245	14.99	539
BRICK	105	8.41	5.320	6.59	159
MONTEREY	106	8.58	5.405	6.94	170
CARAWAY	107	8.28	5.269	7.14	196
SWISS	108	7.88	5.040	7.63	20
ROMANO	110	7.64	4.852	9.02	406
FONTINA	110	8.83	5.442	7.26	227
HARD PARMESAN	111	7.32	4.652	10.14	390
COLBY	112	9.10	5.732	6.74	171
CHEDDAR	114	9.40	5.980	7.06	176
GRATED PARMESAN	122	8.11	4.905	10.9	433
COTTAGE CHEESE, 2%	163	2.31	1.458	28	918
PART SKIM RICOTTA	171	9.81	6.109	14.12	123
COTTAGE CHEESE, lg curd	206	9.03	3.608	23.35	764
WHOLE MILK RICOTTA	216	16.10	10.286	13.96	104
COTTAGE CHEESE, sm curd	220	9.68	3.866	25.02	819

CHICKEN & CHICKEN ENTREES

"Chicken nuggets." One would assume that means said nugget is primarily chicken meat, no? But a study of nuggets from a couple of fast food chains published in the American Journal of Medicine *in 2013 were analyzed microscopically and . . . well, let the researchers tell it: "Striated muscle (chicken meat) was not the predominate component in either nugget. Fat was present in equal or greater quantities along with epithelium [skin], some nerve, and connective tissue. Chicken nuggets are mostly fat and their name is a misnomer."*

Imagine you climbed into a time machine and teleported back to 1984. Which aspect of today's culture would be hardest to explain to denizens of that era?

- The most popular R&B singer in the world will be Alan Thicke's son.
- Career-destroying photos of congressmen will still surface, but they'll mostly be taken by the congressmen themselves.
- Young, hip, sophisticated urbanites will start keeping chickens in their backyards.

In truth, they all seem pretty incredible from the viewpoint of the Big '80s. But it's the trend toward chicken culture that may be the most bizarre. It's a sign of how confusing and concerning our food supply has become that people think it's easier to build a coop off the patio than it is to buy the right eggs. Let's see if we can keep you eating healthy—without being awakened by a rooster.

Let's just call it what it really is: Hefty Man. Mojo-killing trans fats, in the form of partially hydrogenated soybean oil, appears 8 times on the ingredient list, along with propylene glycol, which is something Hefty Man adds to his car engine to keep it from freezing up. Seriously.

WORST SUPERMARKET CHICKEN

Hungry-Man Selects Classic Fried Chicken

970 calories
59 g fat
20 g sat fat
1,480 mg sodium
3 g fiber
13 g sugar
49 g protein

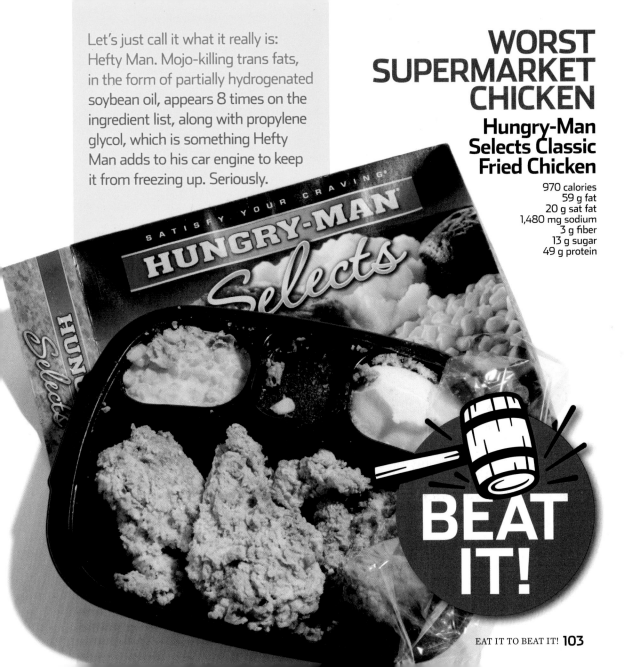

SATISFY YOUR CRAVING

HUNGRY-MAN *Selects*

BEAT IT!

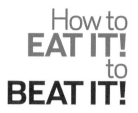

How to
EAT IT!
to
BEAT IT!

It's a mystery how the word "chicken" came to be associated with fear. But its no mystery how the food chicken began striking fear into the hearts of the hungry. From e-coli scares on the 11 o'clock news to the super-crispy, super-greasy concoctions coming out of our fast-food kitchens, chicken is a classic Good Food Gone Bad.

THE CHICKEN RULES

KNOW YOUR MSG. Monosodium glutamate is the ingredient that gives Chinese food its reputation for causing Hunan Hangover. But few packaged goods nowadays include these words, because people are so sensitive to it. Instead, you'll find sources of MSG in lots of packaged chicken products, hidden under natural sounding names: hydrolyzed vegetable protein, autolyzed yeast, hydrolyzed yeast, yeast extract, soy extracts, and protein isolate.

GO ORGANIC. A recent study comparing conventional, antibiotic-free, and USDA organic chicken found that inorganic arsenic concentrations were four times higher in conventional chicken meat than in USDA organic chicken. Organic isn't always worth it, but in the poultry section it is.

STOP EATING PASTE. "Mechanically separated chicken." What could that possibly be? I can't say it any better than the USDA: It's "a paste-like and batter-like poultry product produced by forcing bones with attached edible tissue through a sieve or similar device under high pressure to separate bone from the edible tissue." That's not fowl, that's foul.

HOW TO READ A CHICKEN

*Since chicken is the go-to choice for consumers worried about
their own health and the planet's, more and more chicken producers
have started adding appealing, socially conscious terms to their labels.
Here's what those labels really mean—and what they don't.*

NO HORMONES OR STEROIDS ADDED

 You'll often see this on "natural" chicken products. But hormones and steroids are never given to chickens—it's illegal. So, paying more for chickens marketed as "hormone free" is like paying more for water marked "wet."

BASTED OR SELF-BASTED OR ENHANCED

The chicken meat has been injected with some kind of seasoning solution containing fats, broth, or water. Boneless chicken can be up to 8 percent solution.

CAGE FREE

 Chickens aren't really raised in cages. They're raised in large confinement houses, packed from wall to wall with hens. It's like poultry prison.

FREE RANGE OR FREE ROAMING

 To qualify for this label, the birds must be allowed "access to the outside," but that can mean a few square feet of sunlit concrete for a whole warehouse full of birds. Look instead for the term "pastured" or "pasture-raised," which means they actually got out and stretched their legs.

NATURAL

There's been no artificial ingredients or color added to the meat.

100% VEGETARIAN DIET

The chickens have been fed a diet of grains, without the use of any animal by-products to fatten them up. While it's nice to know they haven't been turned into cannibals, chickens naturally eat grass and insects, not corn and soy. Grains produce fatter, less healthy chickens.

NO ANTIBIOTICS

Farmers must prove that none have been given to the birds, so this is a good term to look for.

BEWARE THE PATTY AND THE NUGGET. Chicken patties and nuggets are often held together with soy protein, corn starch, "flavor," and sugar, and varying amounts of MSG. If you must have a breaded product, go for chicken fingers.

DON'T CLEAN YOUR CHICKEN. Rinsing raw chicken before cooking it can spread harmful bacteria in a 2- to 3-foot radius around your sink. Just cook the chicken to the proper temperature (an internal temperature of 165 degrees) and you'll kill anything you might have wanted to wash off.

THE CHICKEN ADVANTAGE

Lose Weight
Chicken meat is chock-full of quality protein that can help you lose weight and stay satiated while keeping your cholesterol in check, according to research in the journal *Nutrition*. Researchers had overweight women participate in a walking program while having white chicken meat as their main source of protein and found that they lost weight and decreased their LDL cholesterol levels after 12 weeks.

WORST RESTAURANT CHICKEN

Cheesecake Factory Chicken and Biscuits

2,262 calories
68 g sat fat
2,866 mg sodium
164 g carbs

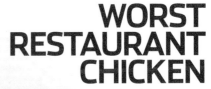

More than a whole day's worth of calories, salt, and fat in one meal. Heads up, Chicken Little: That thud you heard wasn't the sky falling; your doctor just fainted.

BEAT IT!

BEST RESTAURANT CHICKEN

Ruby Tuesday Chicken Bella

Beware the burgers, Mexican fare, and (surprisingly) salads at Ruby Tuesday. But most other entrees are safe bets, especially their Chicken Bella, with 47 grams of protein and 6 grams of fiber for less than 500 calories.

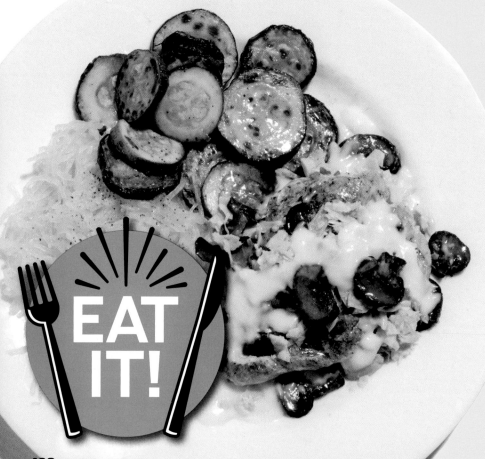

EAT IT!

365 calories
18 g fat
772 mg sodium
3 g fiber
45 g protein

AU BON PAIN
Roasted Mayan Chicken Harvest Rice Bowl
630 calories
16 g fat
4 g sat fat
1,100 mg sodium
3 g fiber
4 g sugar
28 protein

TGI FRIDAY'S
Dragonfire Chicken
660 calories
15 g fat
1.5 g sat fat
2,160 mg sodium
6 g fiber
40 g protein
Sodium is high, but calories are fairly low

RED LOBSTER
Tropical BBQ Glazed Chicken
390 calories
6 g fat
1.5 g sat fat
1,870 mg sodium
27 g protein

ROMANO'S MACARONI GRILL
Grilled Chicken Spiedini
410 calories
11 g fat
2 g sat fat
990 mg sodium
10 g fiber
39 g protein

IHOP
Grilled Balsamic Glazed Chicken
440 calories
22 g fat
3.5 g sat fat
1,060 mg sodium
8 g fiber
13 g sugar
39 g protein

OLIVE GARDEN
Venetian Apricot Chicken
400 calories
7 g fat
2 g sat fat
1,290 mg sodium
6 g fiber
51 g protein

BOSTON MARKET
Rotisserie Chicken Three Piece Dark
390 calories
22 g fat
6 g sat fat
1,270 mg sodium
0 g fiber
<1g sugar
51 g protein

OUTBACK STEAKHOUSE
Grilled Chicken on the Barbie
312 calories
4 g fat
0 g sat fat
869 mg sodium
0 g fiber
10 g sugar
57 g protein

APPLEBEE'S
Sizzling Skillet Chicken Fajitas
1,290 calories
44 g fat
21 g sat fat
4,500 mg sodium
10 g fiber
76 g protein

P.F. CHANG'S
Kung Pao Chicken
1,100 calories
66 g fat
10 g sat fat
2,130 mg sodium
7 g fiber
73 g protein

CHEESECAKE FACTORY
Spicy Cashew Chicken
1,809 calories
7 g sat fat
4,450 mg sodium
252 g carbs

CHILI'S
Honey-Chipotle Chicken Crispers
1,700 calories
77 g fat
13 g sat fat
4,100 mg sodium
13 g fiber
57 g sugar
55 g protein

TGI FRIDAY'S
Hibachi Chicken Skewers
1,330 calories
41 g fat
5 g sat fat
4,760 mg sodium
8 g fiber
56 g protein

FRIENDLY'S
Kickin' Buffalo Chicken Strips
(6 strips)
1,650 calories
116 g fat
16 g sat fat
3,040 mg sodium
8 g fiber
11 g sugar
46 g protein
These buffalo strips deliver 1,040 fat calories!

BEAT IT!

CALIFORNIA PIZZA KITCHEN
Chicken Milanese
1,030 calories
76 g fat
24 g sat fat
1,753 mg sodium
5 g sugar
4 g fiber
70 g protein

ROMANO'S MACARONI GRILL
Chicken Under A Brick
1,440 calories
115 g fat
23 g sat fat
3,640 mg sodium
3 g fiber
76 g protein

IHOP
Fried Chicken Dinner
1,570 calories
84 g fat
24 g sat fat
3,980 mg sodium
6 g fiber
15 g sugar
98 g protein

BEST SUPERMARKET CHICKEN

Kashi Chicken Florentine

290 calories
9 g fat
4.5 g sat fat
550 mg sodium
5 g fiber
1 g sugar
22 g protein

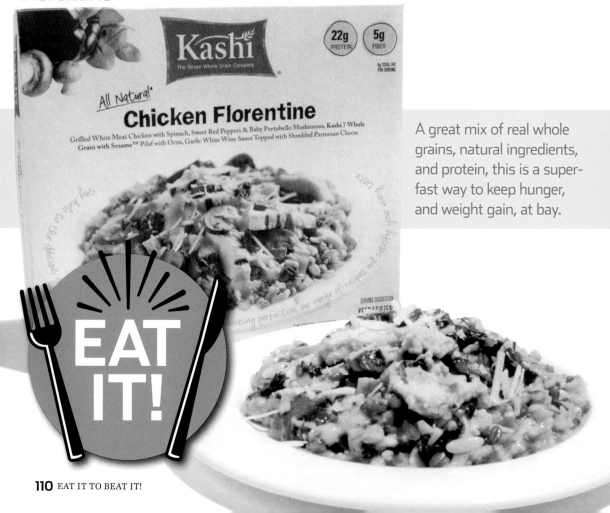

A great mix of real whole grains, natural ingredients, and protein, this is a super-fast way to keep hunger, and weight gain, at bay.

EAT IT!

ATKINS
Chicken Pot Pie, Crustless
330 calories
22 g fat
10 g sat fat
880 mg sodium
3 g fiber
2 g sugar
22 g protein

BLAKE'S
Chicken Pot Pie
310 calories
13 g fat
4 g sat fat
540 mg sodium
2 g fiber
2 g sugar
15 g protein

EVOL BOWLS
Teriyaki Chicken
250 calories
6 g fat
1 g sat fat
490 mg sodium
4 g fiber
8 g sugar
14 g protein

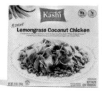

KASHI
Lemongrass Coconut Chicken
300 calories
8 g fat
4 g sat fat
680 mg sodium
7 g fiber
6 g sugar
18 g protein

BANQUET
Chicken Pot Pie
370 calories
21 g fat
8 g sat fat
1,040 mg sodium
3 g fiber
3 g sugar
10 g protein

Mechanically separated chicken, MSG (autolyzed yeast extract)

MARIE CALLENDER'S
Chicken Pot Pie
380 calories
21 g fat
8 g sat fat
740 mg sodium
4 g fiber
4 g sugar
11 g protein

Their "White Meat Chicken" contains chicken mixed with isolated soy protein product, which is isolated soy protein, modified potato starch, corn starch, carrageenan, and soy lecithin. Also contains MSG (autolyzed yeast extract), and methylcellulose (wood pulp). Also, this pie serves two, so double everything you see on the nutrition panel if you eat the whole thing.

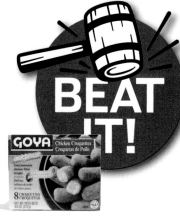

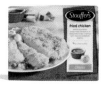

GOYA
Chicken Croquettes
280 calories
12 g fat
2 g sat fat
520 mg sodium
3 g fiber
6 g sugar
13 g protein

Mechanically separated chicken, trans fats (partially hydrogenated soybean and/or cottonseed oil), salt, MSG (monosodium glutamate)

STOUFFER'S
Homestyle Classics Fried Chicken
360 calories
12 g fat
4 g sat fat
800 mg sodium
0 g fiber
7 g sugar
18 g protein

Trans fats (partially hydrogenated soybean and/or cottonseed oil), MSG (yeast extract)

CHINESE FOOD

Ever since Italy coopted their noodle invention, slapped some meatballs on top, and stole all the pasta glory, China has been getting the wrong end of the culinary chopstick. But it wasn't until Chinese food immigrated to America that something truly horrible happened: China's naturally healthy, high-nutrient, flavorful cuisine got loaded up with so much fat, sugar, and monosodium glutamate that we even had to come up with a name for the crappy, headachy way you sometimes feel after eating it: Chinese Restaurant Syndrome.

And the rise of the all-you-can-eat Chinese buffet has only made things worse. A recent study by the good folks at the USDA Human Nutrition Research Center on Aging found the veggie, rice, chicken, and noodle concoctions served up at Chinese restaurants average (that's right, average) 1,474 calories. That's nearly the amount of calories a woman should eat in an entire day, and that's before dessert.

And that's too bad, because Chinese food is loaded with a ton of healthy vegetables, protein, and fiber. You just need to know how to eat around the pitfalls so your fortune cookie doesn't read "For God's sake, don't eat this cookie!"

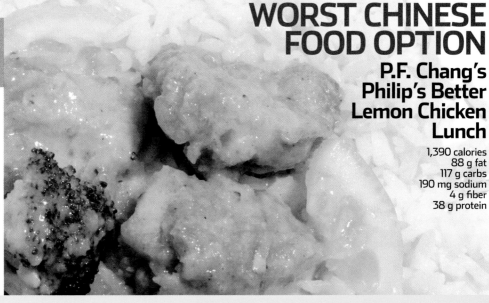

WORST CHINESE FOOD OPTION

P.F. Chang's Philip's Better Lemon Chicken Lunch

1,390 calories
88 g fat
117 g carbs
190 mg sodium
4 g fiber
38 g protein

Perhaps it should be called the "Better Not Eat This" Chicken. This "lunch" option gives you 70 percent of your daily calories and 137 percent of your recommended daily fat intake. You weren't planning on quitting eating at 1 p.m., were you?

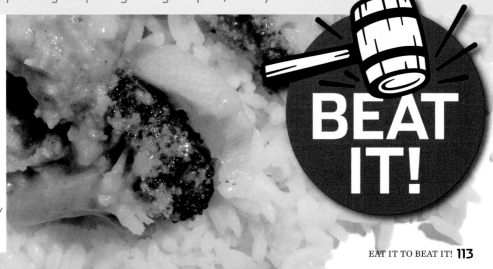

found is P.F. Chang's Sichuan-Style Asparagus. Chang's had this listed as 260 calories. Sounds good for a nice side dish of green vegetables and a little flavor, but the researchers measured it at 558 calories. P.F. Chang's were off by only 115 percent . . . but who's counting?

BEAT IT!

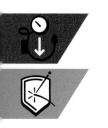

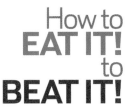

How to
EAT IT!
to
BEAT IT!

Your dim sum joint can be like one of those Chinese finger traps—you reach in, and then you can't pull yourself away. The perfect combination of salt, fat, and sugar coating, those seemingly healthy broccoli dishes are like flypaper for our tastebuds. Here's how to avoid getting Shanghai'd.

THE CHINESE FOOD RULES

VEG OUT. Choose foods that are mostly vegetables, and ask for extra! Make sure those vegetables are brightly colored and crisp (not dark and flimsy). Lightly steamed vegetables have more nutrient value than heavily cooked versions.

HAVE FUN. MEI FUN! This light rice noodle dish can save you hundreds of calories if you choose it instead of greasy lo mein noodles.

FORTUNE COOKIE BREAKDOWN

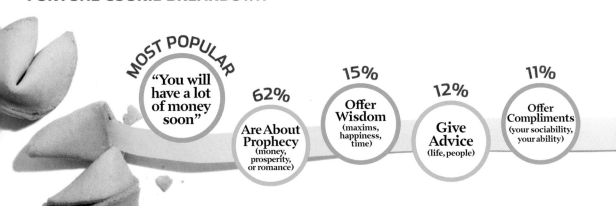

MOST POPULAR

"You will have a lot of money soon"

62% Are About Prophecy (money, prosperity, or romance)

15% Offer Wisdom (maxims, happiness, time)

12% Give Advice (life, people)

11% Offer Compliments (your sociability, your ability)

STICK UP FOR YOURSELF. Using chopsticks while you eat will help you consume fewer calories. Plus, it will give you an air of international sophistication, or at least something to play air drums with.

SKIP THE SAUCES. If the food at Chinese restaurants isn't flavorful enough, you might want to check to make sure your taste buds still work. Plus, those salty sauces add some major milligrams of sodium: duck sauce and hot mustard (100 to 200), hoisin sauce (250), soy sauce (1,000).

THE CHINESE FOOD ADVANTAGE

Boost Immunity

Pairing broccoli with foods rich in the enzyme myrosinase, like radishes, watercress, and mustard, increases broccoli's cancer-fighting abilities, according to a study in the *British Journal of Nutrition*. The combination induces an earlier release of sulforaphane, a compound found in cruciferous vegetables that helps prevent cancer.

Lower Blood Pressure

Cooking with sesame oil and rice bran oil has been linked to improvement in cholesterol levels and decreases in blood pressure similar to those seen with the use of calcium channel blockers, according to research presented at the American Heart Association's High Blood Pressure Research 2012 Scientific Sessions.

---

5 HABITS OF HIGHLY OVERWEIGHT PEOPLE

How normal weight vs obese people approach a Chinese food buffet:

NORMAL WEIGHT:
sits in a booth facing away from the buffet

OBESE:
sits at a table facing the buffet

NORMAL WEIGHT:
browses the selection before choosing food

OBESE:
starts putting food on their plate right away without browsing

NORMAL WEIGHT:
uses chopsticks, puts a napkin on lap

OBESE:
uses fork, no napkin on lap

NORMAL WEIGHT:
15 chews per bite

OBESE:
12 chews per bite

NORMAL WEIGHT:
leaves food on plate

OBESE:
no food left on plate

According to a study in the journal Obesity

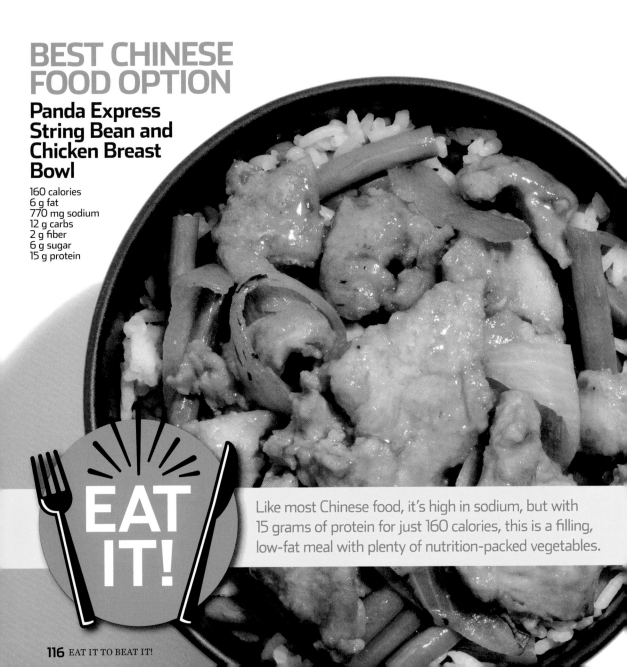

BEST CHINESE FOOD OPTION

Panda Express String Bean and Chicken Breast Bowl

160 calories
6 g fat
770 mg sodium
12 g carbs
2 g fiber
6 g sugar
15 g protein

EAT IT!

Like most Chinese food, it's high in sodium, but with 15 grams of protein for just 160 calories, this is a filling, low-fat meal with plenty of nutrition-packed vegetables.

PANDA EXPRESS

Broccoli Beef
690 calories
40 g fat
57 g carbs
890 mg sodium
4 g fiber
25 g sugar
26 g protein

Shanghai Angus Steak
220 calories
7 g fat
910 mg sodium
19 g carbs
1 g fiber
13g sugar
21 g protein

Mushroom Chicken
180 calories
9 g fat
840 mg sodium
10 g carbs
1 g fiber
4 g sugar
14 g protien

P.F. CHANG'S

Buddha's Feast Vegetarian Plate
(steamed)
260 calories
4 g fat
300 mg sodium
32 g carbs
10 g fiber
26 g protein

P.F. CHANG'S

Fried Rice
All of P.F. Chang's fried rice meals, including even their vegetable fried rice, are over 1,000 calories, with over 2,000 mg of sodium . . . take your pick.

Kung Pao Chicken
1,100 calories
66 g fat
2,130 mg sodium
56 g carbs
7 g fiber
73 g protein

Shrimp with Candied Walnuts
1,380 calories
104 g fat
1,830 mg sodium
74 g carbs
14 g fiber
39 g protein

Ma Pa Tofu
1,030 calories
70 g fat
3,450 mg sodium
44 g carbs
6 g fiber
60 g protein

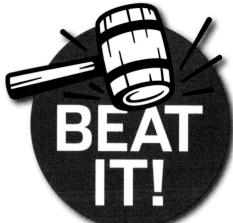

APPLEBEE'S

Crispy Orange Chicken
1,520 calories
49 g fat
2,530 mg sodium
208 g carbs
12 g fiber
64 g protein

Oriental Chicken Rollup
1,190 calories
62 g fat
3,290 mg sodium
125 g carbs
6 g fiber
35 g protein

Oriental Grilled Chicken Salad, Regular
1,290 calories
81 g fat
2,190 mg sodium
90 g carbs
10 g fiber
56 g protein

TGI FRIDAY'S

Hibachi Chicken Skewers
1,330 calories
41 g fat
187 g carbs
4,760 mg sodium
8 g fiber
56 g protein

Hibachi Steak Skewers
1,390 calories
53 g fat
186 g carbs
3,840 mg sodium
8 g fiber
42 g protein

DARK CHOCOLATE

What if a bunch of studies came out proving that something you've always thought was bad for you—drinking coconut rum, or smoking Cuban cigars, or watching *Duck Dynasty* marathons—could actually reduce your risk of heart disease, boost your immune system, and even improve your brain function?

First, there'd be a lot of drunk, smoky, bearded guys in waders walking around. It would be like a Mumford & Sons concert in the Okefenokee.

And second—in about as long as it takes to spell o-p-p-o-r-t-u-n-i-t-y—all the liquor companies, cigar manufacturers, and wader makers would be labeling their product "coconut," "Cuban," or "perfect for ducks"!

Well, that's exactly what's happened to the world of chocolate. Thanks to the naturally occurring nutrients in cocoa beans, studies have linked dark chocolate to everything from boosting your mood to reducing your risk of stroke. Which is why suddenly, everything from candy bars to ice cream to cookies is labeled "dark chocolate."

Must be healthy, right? Pass the cigars!

But wait: Things are murkier than they appear.

Looking for the much-touted health benefits of dark chocolate? You won't find them here. Hershey's doesn't reveal how much heart-healthy cacao goes into their "dark" chocolate, but it doesn't matter anyway: This bar uses "alkalized,"

WORST "DARK" CHOCOLATE
Hershey's Special Dark

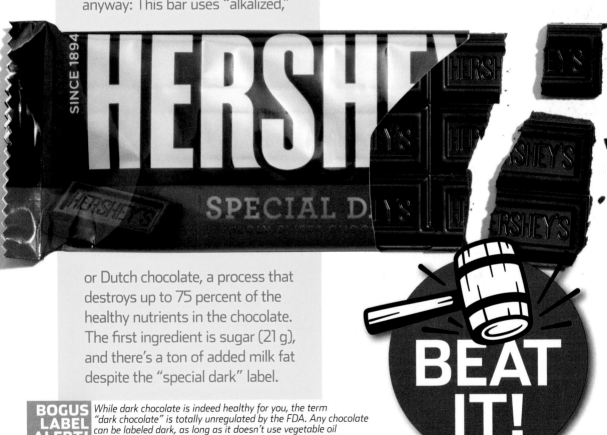

or Dutch chocolate, a process that destroys up to 75 percent of the healthy nutrients in the chocolate. The first ingredient is sugar (21 g), and there's a ton of added milk fat despite the "special dark" label.

BOGUS LABEL ALERT! *While dark chocolate is indeed healthy for you, the term "dark chocolate" is totally unregulated by the FDA. Any chocolate can be labeled dark, as long as it doesn't use vegetable oil as an ingredient. Manufacturers who are serious about their health claims will list the cacao percentage on the label.*

BEAT IT!

How to
EAT IT!
to
BEAT IT!

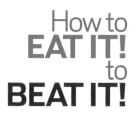

Chocolate's healing properties stem from its key ingredient: cocoa or, as it's properly known, cacao. Chocolatiers (is that a cool job title, or what?) start with cacao beans, which are harvested from the fruit of a cacao tree and are packed with disease-fighting substances, called polyphenols. First, the beans are heated to at least 250 degrees. After roasting, the beans are deskinned and then ground. The heat from the grinding actually liquifies the deskinned beans into what's called chocolate liquor, which is then cooled and pressed to separate the solids from the oils, called cocoa butter. To get cocoa powder, the remaining solids are made into cakes and ground. Even after all that processing, cocoa powder still has more antioxidant power than blueberries, strawberries, and even spinach!

That's why cocoa and, thus, chocolate and hot cocoa drinks have been described as potential medicines dating all the way back to seventeenth-century Europe. More recently, scientists have zeroed in on the substances that make chocolate a healthy food: procyanidins and flavonols, which are specific types of plant polyphenols.

Have you ever tasted a whole cacao bean or, for that matter, unsweetened cocoa powder? Unfortunately, despite their incredible health-giving properties, neither of these taste very good. In fact, completely untouched cacao beans are so bitter they're practically inedible. That's why after the beans are processed into cocoa liquor, cocoa butter, and powder, chocolatiers get to work to mix the polyphenol-rich by-products with sugar, vanilla, and emulsifiers to make chocolate. That doesn't mean you can't find healthy chocolate, it just means you can't justify a daily Snickers bar.

THE CHOCOLATE RULES

SCORE 70 OR ABOVE. What you're looking for is dark chocolate that is at least 70 percent cacao or cocoa. The good stuff, the polyphenols, are what gives cacao its dark color and bitter taste, so the thinking is that the more dark and more bitter you can handle, the more benefits you'll get.

STAY PURE. If you want belly-busting, health-boosting benefits, stick with bars that are just chocolate and nothing else—no marshmallow fluff, cookies 'n' creme, or peanut butter, which only add calories.

DROP THE SUGAR. Look for bars with less than 15 grams of sugar per serving.

WATCH THE CHEAT WORDS. The fat in real chocolate is cocoa butter, which is mainly comprised of hearth-healthy stearic acid. In the U.S., manufacturers can't label a product "chocolate" if they use a vegetable oil other than cocoa butter. Beat It if it's labeled "made with chocolate," "chocolaty," or "chocolate-coating."

DON'T GO DUTCH. Forget anything that's labeled "dutch processed" or "alkalized." Dutch processing means that an alkalizing agent has been added to the cocoa to balance the natural acidity of cacao, which results in a milder taste and, consequently, reduces the flavonol content. A study financed and published by The Hershey Company found that "lightly dutched" and "medium dutched" cocoa destroyed 60 and 77 percent, respectively, of the healthy flavonols.

VALENTINE'S NIGHT

Studies suggest that cocoa flavonols promote production of nitric oxide in the body, which lowers blood pressure by causing the blood vessels to open wider. What else promotes the production of nitric oxide? Hands? If you said "Viagra," you win!

THE CHOCOLATE ADVANTAGE

 ### Lose Weight

Animal studies have shown that cocoa polyphenols may be able to prevent obesity by effecting the way fat is metabolized: A 2011 study published in the *Journal of the Academy of Nutrition and Dietetics* found that overweight and obese women on a reduced-fat diet still lost weight when they allowed themselves a daily dark chocolate snack.

 ### Boost Immunity

A 2008 study in *The Journal of Nutritional Biochemistry* showed that rats fed a cocoa-enriched diet had higher levels of the T-cells and antibodies important for fighting infections.

 ### Improve Mood

A 2013 review of studies in the *British Journal of Clinical Pharmacology* found that flavonols in chocolate improve learning and memory, boost mood and fight emotional stress, and lower the risk of Alzheimer's and stroke.

 ### Lower Blood Pressure

The Kuna Indians of Panama drink 5 cups of flavonol-rich cocoa per day, on average, and incorporate cocoa into many recipes. They also have very little age-related high blood pressure or hypertension, studies have found. A 2008 meta-analysis published in *The American Journal of Clinical Nutrition* found that consuming flavonol-rich cocoa products and dark chocolate reduced the relative risk for stroke mortality by 8 percent.

Lower Cholesterol

A systematic review published in 2006 in the journal *Nutrition & Metabolism* found that cocoa and chocolate reduce cardiovascular risk in many ways, including lowering blood pressure and cholesterol, but also by reducing inflammation, blood clotting, and the hardening of arteries.

Beat Diabetes

In 2011, researchers published a meta-review in *The Journal of Nutrition,* which looked at 24 different studies involving more than 1,100 patients, and concluded that chocolate decreased insulin resistance. More recently, in 2013, a study published in the journal *Diabetic Medicine* found that eating dark chocolate lessened the nasty effects of hyperglycemia or high blood sugar in diabetic patients.

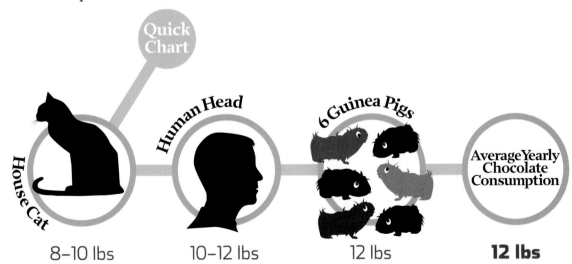

Quick Chart

House Cat
8–10 lbs

Human Head
10–12 lbs

6 Guinea Pigs
12 lbs

Average Yearly Chocolate Consumption
12 lbs

THE BEST DARK CHOCOLATES

Ghirardelli Intense Dark Midnight Reverie

With a whopping 86 percent cacao and a mere 5 g of sugar, Ghirardelli's Intense Dark Midnight Reverie may be the healthiest chocolate bar on the planet.

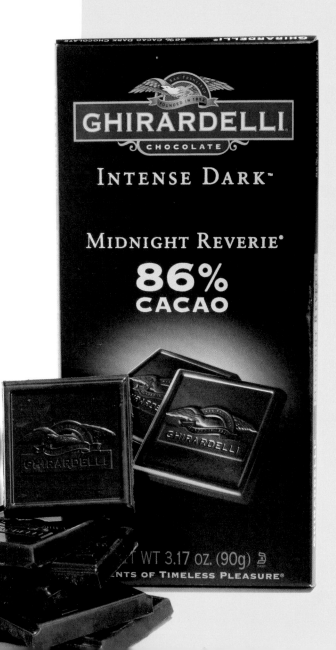

EAT IT!

CHOCOLOVE

Strong Dark Chocolate
70 percent cacao
8 g sugar

Extra Strong Dark Chocolate
77 percent cacao
6 g sugar
Both made with non-GMO soy lecithin

GREEN & BLACK'S ORGANIC

Dark 70%
70 percent cacao
10 g sugar
Non-GMO soy lecithin

Dark 85%
85 percent cacao
8 g sugar

GHIRADELLI

Intense Dark Twilight Delight
72 percent cacao
10 g sugar

TRADER JOE'S

TJ's Pound Plus
72 percent cacao
13 g sugar
Soy lecithin

DAGOBA

New Moon
74 percent cacao
10 g sugar

Eclipse
87 percent cacao
8 g sugar
Both with non-GMO soy lecithin

ENDANGERED SPECIES

Natural Dark Chocolate
72 percent cacao
12 g sugar

Natural Dark Chocolate with Cacao Nibs
72 percent cacao
12 g sugar

Natural Dark Chocolate
88 percent cacao
10 g sugar
All with non-GMO soy emulsifier

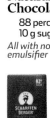

SCHARFFEN BERGER

Extra Dark, Fine Artisan Dark Chocolate
82 percent cacao
8 g sugar

Non-GMO soy lecithin

BEAT IT!

HERSHEY'S

Bliss Dark Chocolate Squares
unspecified cacao percentage not less than 34 percent, processed with alkali
20 g sugar

RUSSELL STOVER

Sugar Free Premium Dark Chocolate
Partially hydrogenated oils (trans fat) and alkalized chocolate

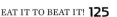

SEE'S CANDIES

Premium Extra Dark Chocolate Bar
62 percent cacao
16 g sugar

DOVE

Silky Smooth Dark Chocolate Bar
unspecified cacao percentage, semisweet, not less than 34 percent
19 g sugar

CONDIMENTS

Imagine a world without squirting mustard, splattering ketchup, or slathering mayo. It would be a bland world, a vast culinary wasteland desperate for flavor. (It would also be a world with much lower dry-cleaning bills, but that's beside the point.)

Condiments put the wag in your hot dog, the TLC in your BLT. And while most of us think of them as having little nutritional impact, the fact is that most condiments actually add significant health benefits to most anything they're spread upon. Mayo has heart-healthy monounsaturated fats, ketchup is long on cancer-busting lycopene, and mustard is a known anti-inflammatory agent. The key is to find packaged goods that are as close to the original recipes as possible.

MAYONNAISE

Although it has a lot more calories per serving than ketchup, mayonnaise is actually a healthier option (in moderation, of course). Because of the oil, mayo is loaded with heart-healthy monounsaturated and polyunsaturated fatty acids (aka MUFAs and PUFAs). And there's no reason to fear the eggs, either.

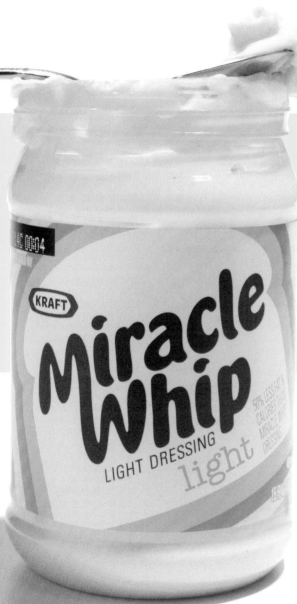

WORST CONDIMENT
Miracle Whip Light

Miracle Whip was the Frankenstein monster of condiments, turning heart-healthy mayonnaise into a festival of sugar, salt, and preservatives. But then came Bride of Frankenstein: Miracle Whip Light. While it does have fewer calories than regular mayo, the folks at Kraft have performed the "miracle" of removing all of the heart-healthy monounsaturated fats of real mayonnaise while boosting the sodium content. The first ingredient is water, with high fructose corn syrup, sugar, and sucralose also on the ingredient list.

20 calories
1.5 g fat
1 g sugar
125 mg sodium

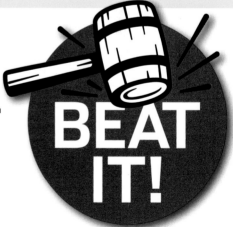

BEAT IT!

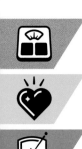
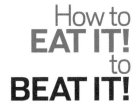

How to
EAT IT!
to
BEAT IT!

Multiple studies have debunked the myth that the dietary cholesterol in egg yolks can harm your heart. Plus, the fat content in mayo helps you absorb the essential fat-soluble vitamins A, D, E, and K in vegetables when you eat mayo with salads and sandwiches.

THE MAYO RULE:

GET FAT. Monounsaturated fats are found in avocados, olives, sunflower seeds, and other things you're probably not eating on a regular basis. So the best thing you can do is look for the oils that provide your body with monos. That's where mayo comes in. A full-fat mayo will have 2 or more grams of the good stuff; avoid anything that's "light," which just means "light on nutrition." In most cases, manufacturers have just taken out the good fats and filled the jar with sugars and starches.

THE MAYO CLINIC

Want another reason to pick real mayonnaise over the phony, reduced-fat versions? Just look at how much money you could save on shaving cream, WD-40, and medicinal shampoos if you have this delicious condiment in your fridge. Here's how to use mayo for fun and profit.

SHAVE YOUR LEGS. The oils in the mayo will leave you with that silky smooth, eggy feeling.

KILL HEAD LICE. Slather your head in mayo, then wear a shower cap to bed. Note: Do not plan on getting lucky tonight.

POLISH YOUR PLANTS. Florists use this trick to make their plants look shiny and fresh.

FIX A SQUEAKY DOOR. The oil in the mayo will help the hinge swing freely.

REMOVE OLD BUMPER STICKERS. It's great that your kid was an honors student. In 1997.

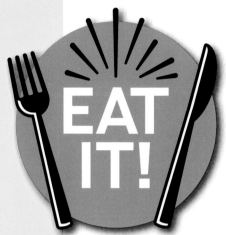

EAT IT!

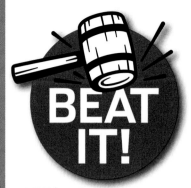

BEAT IT!

KRAFT
Mayo
- 90 calories
- 10 g fat
- 2.5 g mono-unsaturated fat
- 70 mg sodium

HELLMAN'S
Canola Cholesterol Free
- 40 calories
- 4 g fat
- 2 g monounsaturated fat
- 115 mg sodium

A study presented at the American Heart Association's 2013 Scientific Sessions showed that canola oil may help trim belly fat better than other oils.

HELLMAN'S
Real Mayo
- 90 calories
- 10 g fat
- 2.5 g mono-unsaturated fat
- 90 mg sodium

HELLMAN'S
Light Mayo
- 35 calories
- 3.5 g fat
- 1 g monounsaturated fat
- 125 mg sodium

To save a mere 55 calories, why cut down on heart-healthy fats and add 30 percent more sodium?

KRAFT
Mayo with Olive Oil
- 35 calories
- 3 g fat
- 2 g monounsaturated fat
- 1 g sugar
- 95 mg sodium

The Tolstoy-like ingredients list gives us pause, especially when it lists a lot of things not normally found in mayonnaise, like maltodextrin (a form of sugar), lactic acid, potassium sorbate, phosphoric acid, and other yummy-sounding food-like substances.

MIRACLE WHIP
- 40 calories
- 3.5 g fat
- 1 g monounsaturated fat
- 100 mg sodium
- 1 g sugar

Includes three forms of sugar. If chemical experiments like this were really "miracles," they should canonize that guy from Breaking Bad.

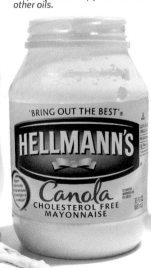

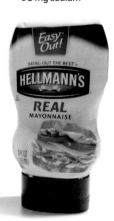

KETCHUP

Back in the 1980s, the Reagan administration caught a lot of flack for trying to categorize ketchup as a vegetable in school lunches. But research seems to indicate that idea wasn't as wacky as it first seemed. Traditionally, ketchup is made from tomatoes, vinegar, salt, pepper, and other spices. Because tomatoes are rich in a nutrient called lycopene (which is found in other red foods like watermelon), it is a powerful health booster.

BEST KETCHUP

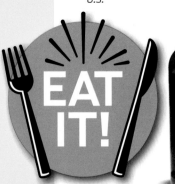

TRADER JOE'S
15 calories
150 mg sodium
2 g sugar

Purely organic, and lower in sugar than most any brand you can find, this is as healthy as any ketchup widely available in the U.S.

MUIR GLEN ORGANIC TOMATO KETCHUP
20 calories
230 mg sodium
3 g sugar

Organic, yes, but slightly higher in calories, sugar, and sodium than our top choices

GREEN WAY
15 calories
150 mg sodium
2 g sugar

Another organic, low-sugar option

ORGANICVILLE ORGANIC KETCHUP
15 calories
125 mg sodium
4 g sugar

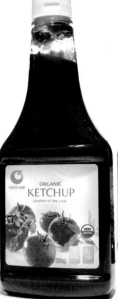

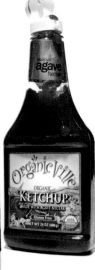

THE KETCHUP RULES

GO ORGANIC. Many times, the word "organic" doesn't necessarily mean the product is healthier. But for ketchup it may actually be worth it. A study published in the *Journal of Agricultural and Food Chemistry* found that organic tomatoes, as well as organic ketchup and tomato juice, had higher levels of disease-fighting antioxidants.

DON'T BE SO SWEET. Almost every ketchup sold in America has sugar or high fructose corn syrup. Try to lower your intake of this non-essential ingredient.

HUNT'S KETCHUP

20 calories
160 mg sodium
4 g sugar

Back in 2010, Hunt's announced it was going to remove high fructose corn syrup from all of its ketchups, but it added it back just two years later.

365 EVERY-DAY VALUE
(WHOLE FOODS)

20 calories
160 mg sodium
4 g sugar

We like the organic ingredients, but there's no reason why this product needs so much sugar, organic or not.

HUNT'S 100% NATURAL KETCHUP
(NO HCFS ADDED)

20 calories
190 mg sodium
4 g sugar

Hunt's now has a special edition in which they've stripped out all the corn syrup, but added in plain sugar.

HEINZ REDUCED SUGAR

5 calories
170 mg sodium
1 g sugar

It is nice to see that Heinz offers a Reduced Sugar product. But it is still sweetened with sucralose.

WORST KETCHUP

ANNIE'S ORGANIC KETCHUP

15 calories
170 mg sodium
4 g sugar

Another organic offering that's higher in sugar than other options

HEINZ KETCHUP

20 calories
160 mg sodium
4 g sugar

Contains both sugar and high fructose corn syrup

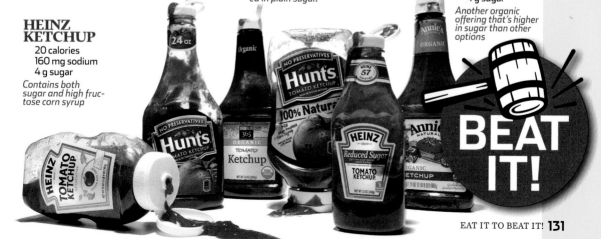

BEAT IT!

MUSTARD

The tangy yellow paste you know from the ballpark is derived from the seeds of the mustard plant. Mustard has anti-inflammatory properties and is extremely low in calories. So low, in fact, most brands can list zero calories/per serving.

THE MUSTARD RULE

DON'T CALL ME HONEY. Most honey mustards use different forms of sugar, with only a hint of honey. If you want honey mustard, do this: Take some mustard. Take some honey. Mix. See how simple?

BEST MUSTARDS

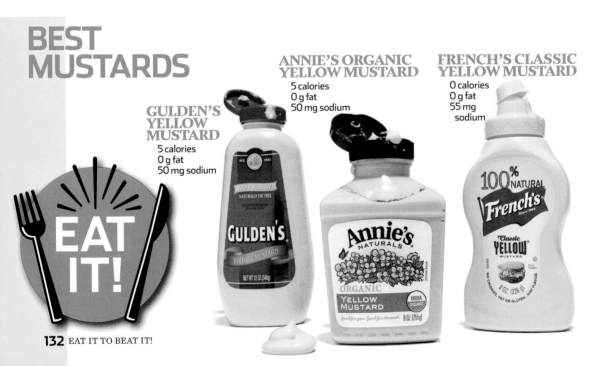

GULDEN'S YELLOW MUSTARD
5 calories
0 g fat
50 mg sodium

ANNIE'S ORGANIC YELLOW MUSTARD
5 calories
0 g fat
50 mg sodium

FRENCH'S CLASSIC YELLOW MUSTARD
0 calories
0 g fat
55 mg sodium

EAT IT!

THE CONDIMENT ADVANTAGE

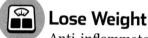
Lower Cholesterol

According to a Finnish study from 2007, British people who added ketchup to their breakfast, lunch, and tea saw their LDL drop significantly in just three weeks. (You do take tea, don't you?)

Lose Weight

Anti-inflammatory herbs like those in mustard can only help.

Beat Diabetes

A Mayo clinic paper linked the healthy fats in mayonnaise to a decreased risk for diabetes.

Boost Immunity

The phytonutrient lycopene is linked to a lower risk of some forms of cancer.

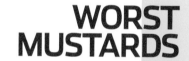

WORST MUSTARDS

BOGUS LABEL ALERT!

French's "honey mustard" is sweet and tinted brown. That must be from the honey, right? But, in fact, three forms of sweetener—high fructose corn syrup, sugar, and corn syrup—appear on the label before honey does. Even the honey brown color is fake—it comes from a derivative of carrots.

FRENCH'S HONEY MUSTARD

10 calories
0 g fat
<1 g sugar
35 mg sodium

TASTE REAL HONEY GOODNESS

French's
Honey MUSTARD

NO FAT OR GLUTEN. JUST 10 CALORIES.

12 OZ. (340 g)

GULDEN'S
ZESTY HONEY MUSTARD

NET WT 12 OZ (340g)

GULDEN'S ZESTY HONEY MUSTARD FAT FREE

10 calories
0 g fat
2 g sugar

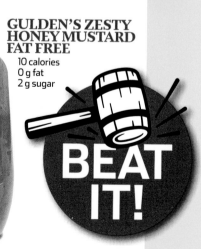

BEAT IT!

COOKIES

I know what you're hoping for. You're hoping that in this chapter, I'll finally reveal the heart-healthy hamantaschen, the muscle-making macaroon, the belly-busting bourbon biscuit. Thin mints that will make you thin, fortune cookies that will bring you good fortune, lady fingers that will fit your lady figure.

Well, that's not going to happen. There's no way to make an Oreo into a health food, even if you dunk it in organic, fat-free, grass-fed milk. But cookies are a dessert, and you ought to reward yourself with a few at night when you're in your jams and settling in for a cozy evening of *Modern Family*. So indulge me in this chapter. Just indulge wisely, and learn to avoid some of the worst cookies on the market.

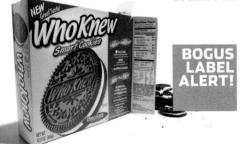

BOGUS LABEL ALERT!

Who Knew Smart Cookies Chocolate Sandwich cookies seem positioned as the healthy alternative to Oreos. "Filled with Good Stuff," says their packaging: whole grains, fiber, and calcium. But a closer look at the ingredients shows that white flour, sugar, and granulated sugar all come before whole grains. While there's a bit more fiber than in an Oreo, the calorie, fat, and sugar counts are nearly identical. It's like saying King Kong is healthier for your city than Godzilla: Neither one of them is going to improve your real estate values.

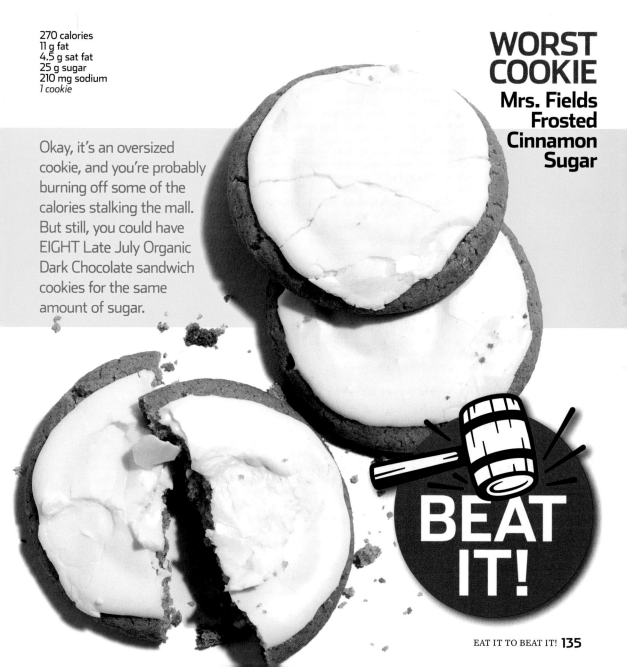

270 calories
11 g fat
4.5 g sat fat
25 g sugar
210 mg sodium
1 cookie

WORST COOKIE

Mrs. Fields Frosted Cinnamon Sugar

Okay, it's an oversized cookie, and you're probably burning off some of the calories stalking the mall. But still, you could have EIGHT Late July Organic Dark Chocolate sandwich cookies for the same amount of sugar.

BEAT IT!

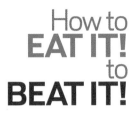

How to EAT IT! to BEAT IT!

Whoever invented the idea of cookies and milk knew what they were doing. Cookies are nothing more than really efficient sugar-delivery systems—filled with empty carbs and no protein or fiber to slow down their absorption. Dunk a cookie in some milk, however, and you've added the missing protein and slowed down the sugar spike that cookies alone will cause. (Just make sure you drink the rest of the milk, even if the crumbs are drifting around the bottom.)

THE COOKIE RULES

THE CREAM IS A NIGHTMARE. Like many prepackaged baked goods, cookies are often loaded with trans fats and saturated fats. But this is especially true of cream-filled versions.

DON'T GET OVERSERVED. One trick marketers use is to play with serving size so as to utterly confuse us hapless cookie lovers. For example, a serving of Chips Ahoy is 33 grams. Dig in! Oh, you don't have your food scale handy? Then how would you know that eating just 4 cookies means you've overserved yourself?

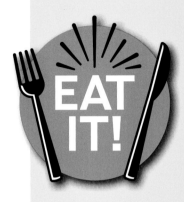

EAT IT!

BEST COOKIE

Kashi Oatmeal Dark Chocolate Soft-Baked Cookie

This whole-grain cookie packs more fiber than your average slice of 100% whole-wheat bread. Whenever you can sneak fiber into an indulgence, you're doing right by your body.

130 calories
5 g fat
1.5 g sat fat
8 g sugar
65 mg sodium
4 g fiber
1 cookie

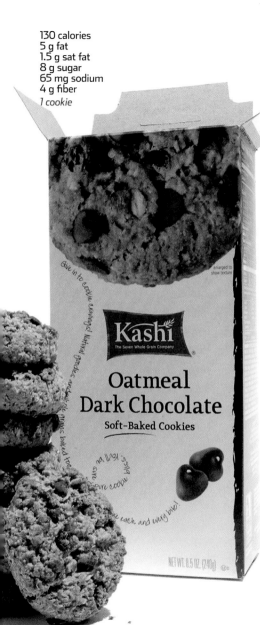

Kashi
The Seven Whole Grain Company

Oatmeal Dark Chocolate

Soft-Baked Cookies

NET WT. 8.5 OZ. (240g)

TATE'S
Whole Wheat Dark Chocolate Cookies

80 calories
4 g fat
2.5 g sat fat
80 g sodium
0 g fiber
5 g sugar
<1 g protein
1 cookie

BEAR NAKED
Soft-Baked Double Chocolate Granola Cookies

130 calories
5 g fat
1 g sat fat
11 g sugar
2 g fiber
1 cookie

A little high in sugar, but half of the fat in this cookie is heart-healthy mono-unsaturated fat

CAVEMAN COOKIES
Original

130 calories
7 g fat
0.5 g sat fat
13 g sugar
1 g fiber
2 cookies

Also a little sugary, but you get 3.5 g of heart-healthy monounsaturated fat and 3 g of protein in a serving

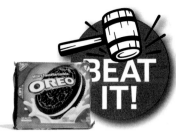

BEAT IT!

OREO

160 calories
7 g fat
2 g sat fat
14 g sugar
1 g fiber
3 cookies

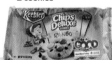

KEEBLER
E.L. Fudge Double Stuffed

180 calories
9 g fat
3.5 g sat fat
13 g sugar
1 g fiber
2 cookies

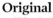

Chips Deluxe Rainbow

160 calories
8 g fat
3 g sat fat
10 g sugar
<1g fiber
2 cookies

The "rainbow" comes from 5 different kinds of artificial coloring and delicious additives like carnauba wax, which you'll also recognize as shoe polish

CRACKERS

You may think of crackers as little more than edible plates, bland diskettes whose only job is to hold the fatty spoils of your stacking and spreading expertise. And in their original form, that's right—crackers were conceived as little more than flour, water, and salt, as bland as a Disney starlet.

But nowadays, crackers have gone the way of Miley Cyrus, getting salty, spicy, and generally tarted up with any number of unsavory ingredients. Which is a bummer, since the whole idea of bland crackers is that we get to besmirch them with our own concoctions—we add the bad stuff. Having a cracker that's pre-loaded with additives is like Kanye West having a microphone that does the trash talking for him. Where's the fun in that?

While the original Ritz has a bit more fat, the Roasted Vegetable version deserves an extra ding for polishing up their health halo by putting "with real vegetables" on the box. They would be just as accurate if they put "with real oxygen" on the package, as there's far more air in the bag than there are vegetables. While dehydrated peppers, tomatoes, and cabbage do show up on the ingredients list, they're preceded, and far outweighed, by white flour, soybean oil, sugar, and partially hydrogenated oil.

160 calories
7 g fat
2 g saturated fat
300 mg sodium
0 g fiber
1 g sugar
10 crackers

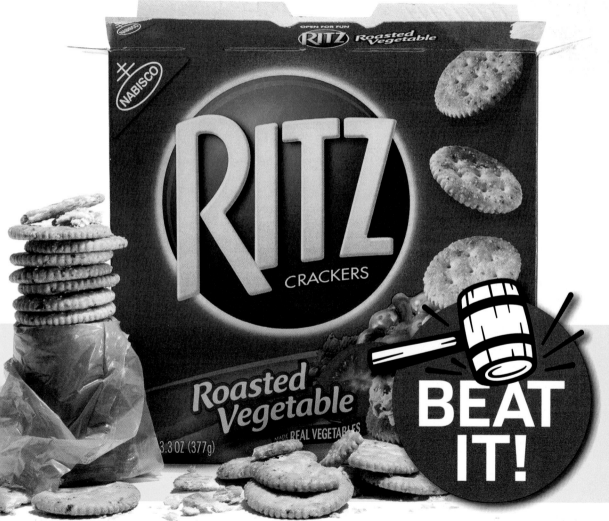

WORST
CRACKER
Ritz Roasted Vegetable

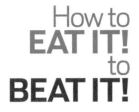

How to
EAT IT!
to
BEAT IT!

Look, you know you're going to put some cheese on that cracker. And maybe some pepperoni. And probably some other delicious bad stuff that makes life worth living. *Eat It to Beat It!* is all about indulging, without some mega-conglomerate food company sabotaging your good, clean, bad-food fun. Here's how.

THE CRACKER RULES

KEEP IT SIMPLE, NOT STUPID. Partially hydrogenated oils, which are industry lingo for trans fats, have been linked to both heart disease and cognitive decline. When you put a slice of

BEST CRACKER

Ak-Mak 100% Whole of the Wheat

110 calories
2g fat
0 g trans fat
223 mg sodium
4 g fiber
0 g sugar
5 crackers

Those of you who enjoy eating your crackers while wearing sandals will like the fact that these are made from organic wheat. But with a gram of protein and nearly a whole gram of fiber in every single cracker, this more than qualifies as a health food.

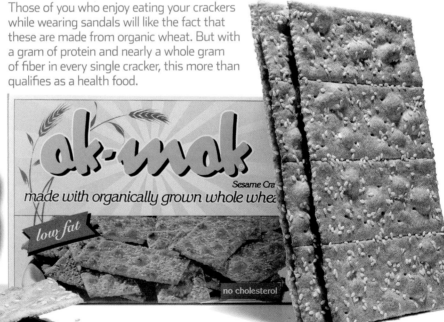

EAT IT!

cheese on top of a cracker that's high in trans fats, it's actually the cracker, not the cheese, that's worse for your health.

BOOST YOUR MORAL FIBER. Take this as an opportunity to sneak fiber into your diet even while eating junk. Look for at least a full gram of fiber per serving.

RETREAT FROM "WHEAT." Most "wheat" crackers are primarily enriched flour, sometimes with caramel coloring to make them look "wheaty." Make sure the first ingredient is "whole wheat flour."

LITTLE FAT, NOT MUCH SUGAR. Follow this rule and every-thing else will fall into place.

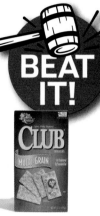

KEEBLER
Club
Crackers
Multi-Grain

120 calories
5 g fat
260 mg
  sodium
0 g fiber
4 g sugar
8 crackers

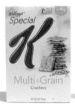

SPECIAL K

Snack Crackers Multi-Grain

40 calories
1 g fat
73 mg sodium
1 g fiber
2 g sugar
8 crackers

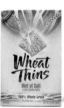

WHEAT THINS

Snacks, Whole Grain, Hint of Salt

150 calories
5 g fat
55 g sodium
3 g fiber
4 g sugar
2 g protein
16 crackers

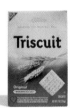

TRISCUIT
Original

120 calories
4.5 g fat
160 mg
  sodium
3 g fiber
0 g sugar
6 crackers

SUNSHINE
Cheez-It Original

50 calories
2.5 g fat
77 mg sodium
0 fiber
0 sugar
9 crackers

NABISCO
Wheat Thins Original

70 calories
2.5 g fat
115 mg sodium
1 g fiber
2 g sugar
8 crackers

CARR'S
Whole Wheat Crackers

320 calories
16 g fat
400 mg
  sodium
4 g fiber
12 g sugar
8 crackers

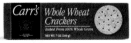

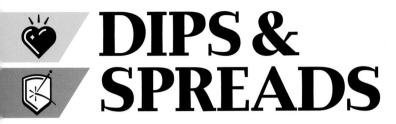

DIPS & SPREADS

Buying a jar of dip in the supermarket is like celebrating Opposite Day, where every product is actually the opposite of what the label says. For example, if the label says "avocado dip," then there's probably very little avocado involved. Similarly, if you're buying a "cheese dip," do not be foolish enough to expect cheese. It's Opposite Day, remember?

Thing is, whatever you're sticking into your dip is probably already bad for you—fried and coated with salt. You could, with some smart shopping, pick out a dip that's healthy enough to help reverse the snack damage. But that would require you to buy the food that's actually mentioned on the label—and that takes a little more hunting than you'd think. Here's where reading the ingredient list really matters.

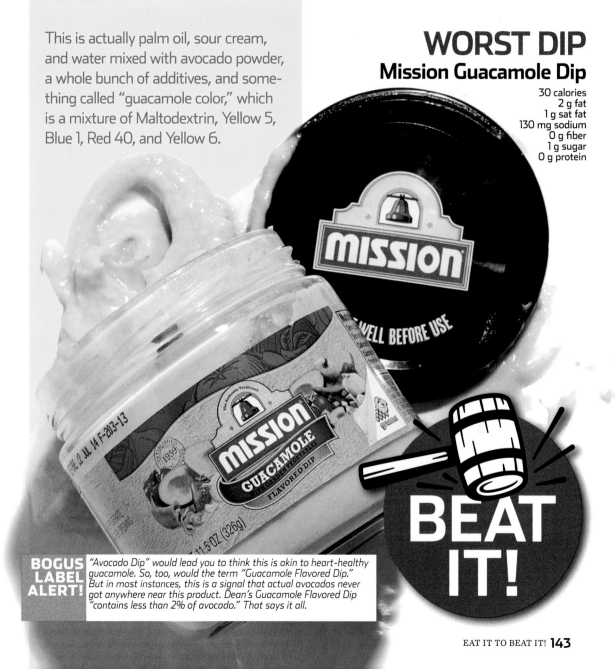

This is actually palm oil, sour cream, and water mixed with avocado powder, a whole bunch of additives, and something called "guacamole color," which is a mixture of Maltodextrin, Yellow 5, Blue 1, Red 40, and Yellow 6.

WORST DIP
Mission Guacamole Dip

30 calories
2 g fat
1 g sat fat
130 mg sodium
0 g fiber
1 g sugar
0 g protein

BOGUS LABEL ALERT! *"Avocado Dip" would lead you to think this is akin to heart-healthy guacamole. So, too, would the term "Guacamole Flavored Dip." But in most instances, this is a signal that actual avocados never got anywhere near this product. Dean's Guacamole Flavored Dip "contains less than 2% of avocado." That says it all.*

BEAT IT!

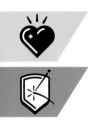

How to EAT IT! to BEAT IT!

THE DIP RULES

USE YOUR BEAN. It's hard to find a bad bean dip; most are low in calories and have a fiber kick.

DON'T DOUBLE THE SALT. Most of what you're dipping is going to be high in sodium already. Choose a dip that's no more than 200 mg per serving.

GET REAL. Real guacamole is made mostly of avocado. Real hummus is made of garbanzo beans. Real salsa con queso is made of cheese. Why is this so hard?

BEST DIP

Amy's Organic Salsa Medium

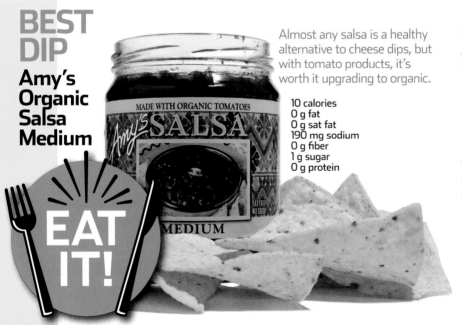

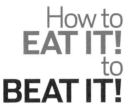

Almost any salsa is a healthy alternative to cheese dips, but with tomato products, it's worth it upgrading to organic.

10 calories
0 g fat
0 g sat fat
190 mg sodium
0 g fiber
1 g sugar
0 g protein

FRITOS
All Natural Bean Dip

35 calories
1 g fat
0 g sat fat
190 mg sodium
2 g fiber
0 sugar
2 g protein

WHOLLY GUACAMOLE
Classic

60 calories
5 g fat
1 g sat fat
105 mg sodium
2 g fiber
0 g sugar
1 g protein

THE DIP ADVANTAGE

Boost Immunity

Garbanzo beans, the central ingredient in hummus, possess bioactive compounds capable of inhibiting the formation of precancerous lesions in mice, so their consumption could contribute to a reduction in colon cancer incidence, according to a study by the University of Illinois.

Lower Cholesterol

Olive oil, garlic, and beans of all types can lower cholesterol.

BEAT IT!

HERDEZ
Salsa Casera, Hot
- 10 calories
- 0 g fat
- 0 g sat fat
- 270 mg sodium
- 0 g fiber
- 0 g protein
- 0 g sugar

SABRA
Chipotle Hummus
- 70 calories
- 4.5 g fat
- 0.5 g sat fat
- 130 mg sodium
- 2 g fiber
- 0 g sugar
- 2 g protein

ATHENOS
Hummus Original
- 50 calories
- 3 g fat
- 0 g sat fat
- 160 mg sodium
- 1 g fiber
- 1 g sugar
- 1 g protein

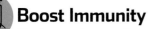

NEWMAN'S OWN
Black Bean & Corn Salsa
- 20 calories
- 0 g fat
- 0g sat fat
- 140 mg sodium
- 2 g fiber
- 1 g sugar
- 1 g protein

PACE
Jalapeno & Pepper Jack
- 50 calories
- 3 g fat
- 1 g sat fat
- 310 mg sodium
- 1 g fiber
- 1 g sugar
- 1 g protein

OKIOS
French Onion Dip
- 25 calories
- 1 g fat
- 0.5 g sat fat
- 160 mg sodium
- 0 g fiber
- 1 g sugar
- 2 g protein

Salsa con Queso
- 40 calories
- 3 g fat
- 0.5 g sat fat
- 200 mg sodium
- 0 g fiber
- 1 g sugar
- 0 g protein

TOSTITOS
Salsa Con Queso
- 40 calories
- 2.5 g fat
- 1 g sat fat
- 280 mg sodium
- <1g fiber
- <1g protein
- <1 g sugar

MARIE'S
Roasted French Onion Dip
- 100 calories
- 10 g fat
- 3 g sat fat
- 220 mg sodium
- 0 g fiber
- 1 g sugar
- 1 g protein

FISH

Fish are confusing.

Was it halibut that you ate last night—or haddock? Was it fluke or flounder? Redfish or whitefish? Bluefin or yellowtail? Snow crab or stone crab? Which one was good for the environment? Which one was good for your heart? And which one was so loaded with mercury it was like chewing on a thermometer?

The only thing we know for certain about seafood is that it's better for you to eat the fish than for the fish to eat you. Beyond that . . . well, let's see if we can't clear up some of the confusion.

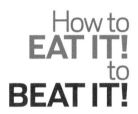

How to
EAT IT!
to
BEAT IT!

The unique health benefits from fish come from the fact that many are loaded with omega-3 fatty acids, which are shown to improve your cholesterol profile and work as natural anti-depressants for the brain. An ideal diet has an equal mix of omega-3 fats and omega-6 fats, which come from corn and other seeds. Unfortunately, today's American diet has up to 25 times as much omega-6 as it does omega-3s, so upping your fish intake would seem like a good idea. But it's more complicated than that.

THE FISH RULES

STAY OFF THE FARM. Farm-raised fish are fed crappy diets of corn and soy, so they're loaded up with inflammation-encouraging omega-6 fatty acids, instead of heart healthy omega-3s. A 2008 report in the *Journal of the American Dietetic Association* found

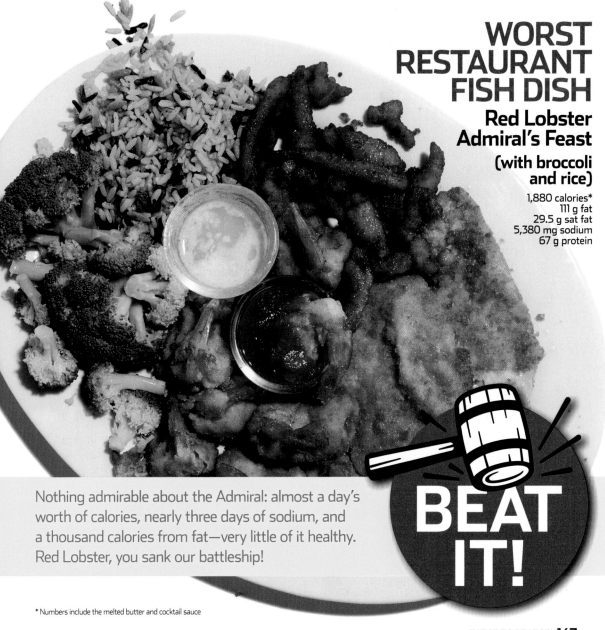

WORST RESTAURANT FISH DISH

Red Lobster Admiral's Feast

(with broccoli and rice)

1,880 calories*
111 g fat
29.5 g sat fat
5,380 mg sodium
67 g protein

Nothing admirable about the Admiral: almost a day's worth of calories, nearly three days of sodium, and a thousand calories from fat—very little of it healthy. Red Lobster, you sank our battleship!

BEAT IT!

* Numbers include the melted butter and cocktail sauce

that eating certain farmed fish, such as tilapia and catfish, may actually harm people suffering from heart disease. And according to Harvard researchers, farmed fish often have up to 10 times more toxins than wild fish.

NIX THE FISH STIX. Breaded and fried fish is further loaded with omega-6 fats. If you're going for a fish fry, at least make sure that fish isn't tilapia or catfish. Haddock, flounder, pollack, hake and cod are all good options.

STAY DRY. Sodium tripolyphosphate (STPP) is a chemical additive that can make spoiled and expired fish seem fresh because it causes the fish to hold onto moisture. It is a suspected neurotoxin, registered pesticide, and air contaminant, yet the FDA considers it "generally recognized as safe" to eat. Because it causes the fish fillets to retain water, it can also make a cut of fish weigh more. Europe, Canada, and other countries have limits on the total level of STPP allowed in seafood (.1 percent to .5 percent), but the U.S. has no such regulations. Companies aren't required to label this additive, but some packaged products do. Seafood labeled as "dry" has not been treated with STPP (you'll see this a lot with scallops and shrimp). Seafood marked as "wet" has been soaked in it.

SAY NO TO CYANIDE. You'll often see the additive disodium EDTA in packaged fish, added to "protect flavor" or "protect

BOGUS LABEL ALERT! *Atlantic salmon. There is no such thing. "Atlantic salmon" is marketing speak for "farm-raised" salmon. A study at the State University of New York recently warned that we should not eat farmed salmon more than twice a month, because the fish are so contaminated with chemicals. Special gross-you-out fact: Because they eat a diet of corn, soy, and fish oil, a farmed salmon's flesh is naturally white, not pink. So anytime you buy Atlantic salmon with that lovely pink color, it's because the farmer bought feed pellets containing synthetic pigments to color the salmon's flesh from the inside out. (Note: Norwegian salmon is another way of saying "farm-raised.")*

250 calories
10 g fat
360 mg sodium
0 g fiber
2 g sugar
29 g protein

WORST SUPERMARKET FISH
Sea Cuisine Parmesan Crusted Tilapia

Farmed tilapia is naturally higher in less-healthy omega-6 fatty acids, and the added white flour and vegetable oils only hurt its nutritional profile more.

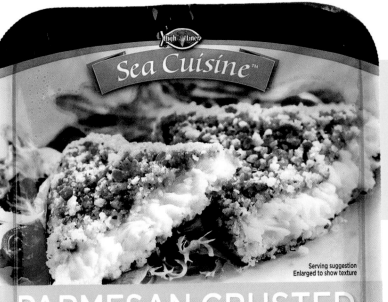

Serving suggestion
Enlarged to show texture

Sea Cuisine™

PARMESAN CRUSTED
TILAPIA

Premium white and flaky Tilapia fillets with Parmesan cheese, Tuscan herbs, and savory breadcrumbs

SERVES 2

GOURMET CRUSTED™

NET WT 10 oz (284g)

BEAT IT!

color." This additive is made from cyanide and formaldehyde. (Sounds appetizing, right?) It has been shown to hinder the body's ability to absorb nutrients.

THE FISH ADVANTAGE

Lower Cholesterol
People with high intakes of omega-3 fatty acids from fish have a decreased risk of coronary heart disease. The American Heart Association recommends that we eat about two meals of fatty fish (wild salmon, herring, sardines) per week.

Lose Weight
Eating fish that are rich in omega-3 fatty acids, like wild salmon, will help you feel full longer because omega-3s increase blood levels of leptin, a hormone that promotes satiety. Also, researchers from Japan have found that eating fish helps you control your weight and gain less abdominal fat because omega-3s increase the enzymes that stimulate fat metabolism.

Improve Mood
Some studies have found that omega-3 fatty acids can improve the effects of antidepressant drugs when the two are taken together. Omega-3s may also protect against age-related cognitive decline.

Boost Immunity
A recent study in the *Journal of Leukocyte Biology* describes that DHA-rich fish oil enhances immune function.

Tears of a Clownfish

A recent study found that fish swimming in waters polluted with anti-anxiety drugs become bold, fearless, asocial, and gluttonous.

THE FISH COUNTER

Here's a glance at the 12 most commonly eaten fish, and which are healthiest for your body—and the Earth—based on omega-3 to omega-6 ratio, toxin levels, and environmental impact.

Wild Alaskan Salmon, Chinook
OMEGA-3: 1,570 mg
OMEGA-6: 238 mg

TOXIN LEVELS	ENVIRO FOOTPRINT
LOW	GOOD

Alaskan Pollack
OMEGA-3: 484 mg
OMEGA-6: 35 mg

TOXIN LEVELS	ENVIRO FOOTPRINT
LOW	GOOD

Atlantic Cod
OMEGA-3: 135 mg
OMEGA-6: 29 mg

TOXIN LEVELS	ENVIRO FOOTPRINT
MODERATE	MODERATE

Clams
OMEGA-3: 248 mg
OMEGA-6: 97 mg

TOXIN LEVELS	ENVIRO FOOTPRINT
LOW	MODERATE

Blue Crab
OMEGA-3: 151 mg
OMEGA-6: 48 mg

TOXIN LEVELS	ENVIRO FOOTPRINT
MODERATE	GOOD

Salmon
(Atlantic Farmed)
OMEGA-3: 1,920 mg
OMEGA-6: 1,648 mg

TOXIN LEVELS	ENVIRO FOOTPRINT
HIGH	BAD

Shrimp
OMEGA-3: 245 mg
OMEGA-6: 219 mg

TOXIN LEVELS	ENVIRO FOOTPRINT
MODERATE	GOOD/BAD*

Canned Tuna
(white, canned in water)
OMEGA-3: 793 mg
OMEGA-6: 90 mg

TOXIN LEVELS	ENVIRO FOOTPRINT
HIGH	GOOD

Canned Tuna
(light, canned in water)
OMEGA-3: 193 mg
OMEGA-6: 141 mg

TOXIN LEVELS	ENVIRO FOOTPRINT
MODERATE	GOOD

Tilapia
OMEGA-3: 156 mg
OMEGA-6: 278 mg

TOXIN LEVELS	ENVIRO FOOTPRINT
LOW	GOOD

Catfish
OMEGA-3: 150 mg
OMEGA-6: 869 mg

TOXIN LEVELS	ENVIRO FOOTPRINT
LOW	GOOD

Pangasius (Basa, an imported catfish also called white roughy)
OMEGA-3: 10 mg
OMEGA-6: 500 mg

TOXIN LEVELS	ENVIRO FOOTPRINT
LOW	BAD

OTHER GOOD OPTIONS AT THE FISH COUNTER > Atlantic mackerel, striped bass, sardines, herring, rainbow trout, flounder

AVOID DUE TO EXTREMELY HIGH MERCURY > swordfish, shark, king mackerel, orange roughy, marlin, ahi tuna, and gulf tilefish

MERCURY FALLING

Drinking green or black tea may keep the toxins in seafood from entering your blood, according to Purdue University researchers. Another study found that drinking tea or coffee with your fish can reduce your body's ability to absorb mercury by 50 to 60 percent.

BEST FAST-FOOD FISH

Long John Silver's Hold the Batter Cod

Most of what's on offer at Long John Silver's is fried and loaded with unhealthy omega-6s. Should you be taken captive and held hostage in one, this is by far the healthiest option.

(1 piece)
45 calories
0 g fat
111 mg sodium
0 fiber
0 sugar
10 g protein

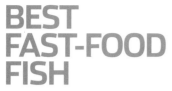

EAT IT!

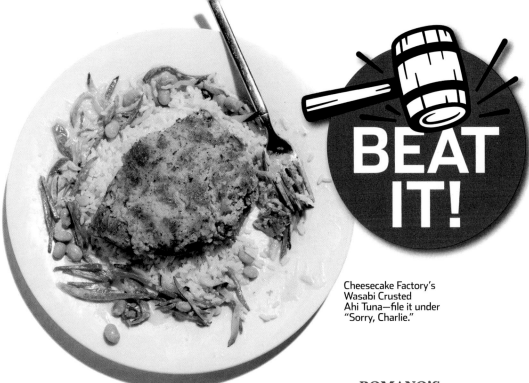

Cheesecake Factory's Wasabi Crusted Ahi Tuna—file it under "Sorry, Charlie."

CHEESECAKE FACTORY
Wasabi Crusted Ahi Tuna
- 1,750 calories
- 58 g sat fat
- 1,300 mg salt
- 113 carbs (as served)

APPLEBEE'S
New England Fish & Chips
- 1,690 calories
- 126 g fat
- 22 g sat fat
- 2,840 mg sodium
- 92 g carbs
- 9 g fiber
- 46 g protein

TGI FRIDAY'S
Jack Daniel's Salmon & Grilled Shrimp Scampi
(with broccoli and rice)
- 1,610 calories
- 72.5 g fat
- 19.5 g sat fat
- 6,400 mg sodium
- 12 g fiber
- 65 g protein

DENNY'S
Fish and Chips
- 1,330 calories
- 73 g fat
- 1,930 mg sodium
- 11 g fiber
- 38 g protein
- 7 g sugar

ROMANO'S MACARONI GRILL
Parmesan-Crusted Sole
- 1,550 calories
- 104 g fat
- 44 g sat fat
- 1,220 mg sodium
- 5 g fiber
- 56 g protein

UNO CHICAGO GRILL
Fish and Chips
- 1,290 calories
- 89 g fat
- 12 g sat fat
- 3,250 mg sodium
- 11 g fiber
- 2 g sugar
- 43 g protein

BEST
SUPERMARKET FISH

Wild Planet Canned Wild Albacore Tuna

120 calories
6 g fat
250 mg sodium
16 g protein

This albacore tuna is pole/troll hand line caught, and these methods catch younger tuna with lower mercury levels. Plus, the can is certified BPA-free. This is the best brand of canned and pouched fish.

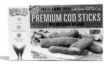

NATURAL SEA
Premium Cod Fish Sticks

190 calories
8 g fat
240 mg sodium
2 g fiber
11 g protein

Premium Cod Fish Fillets

120 calories
5 g fat
200 mg sodium
1 g fiber
6 g protein

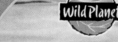

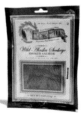

ECHO FALLS
Wild Alaskan Smoked Sockeye Salmon

120 calories
6 g fat
630 mg sodium
0 fiber
15 g protein

Wild Planet

You've never tasted tuna like this before! We hand-cut and pack delicious, premium tuna steaks in a micro-cannery process. All the Omega 3 oils are retained and no liquid is added; please don't drain. We select smaller fish with less mercury accumulation to assure the lowest mercury level available.

Wild Planet packs 100% pure tuna No water, oil or fillers added.

EAT IT!

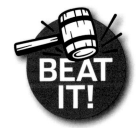
BEAT IT!

HENRY & LISA'S

Wild Alaskan Fish Nuggets

220 calories
9 g fat
360 mg sodium
3 g fiber
13 g protein

Wild Alaskan Salmon Burgers

120 calories
3.5 g fat
210 mg sodium
2 g fiber
14 g protein

CENTO

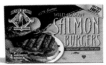

Sardines in Olive Oil

110 calories
6 g fat
370 mg sodium
0 fiber
13 g protein

BUMBLE BEE

Wild Pink Salmon (pouch)

60 calories
1.5 g fat
180 mg sodium
0 fiber
0 g sugar
14 g protein

BAR HARBOR

Whole Maine Cherrystone Clams

45 calories
0.5 g fat
330 mg sodium
0 g fiber
8 g protein

MRS. PAUL'S

Crunchy Fish Sticks

230 calories
10 g fat
480 mg sodium
<1 g fiber
11 g protein

Treated with the pesticide and suspected neurotoxin sodium tripolyphosphate (STPP). (Mrs. Paul's Flounder and Haddock Fillets also have STPP)

GORTON'S

Crunchy Breaded Fish Fillets

250 calories
13 g fat
470 mg sodium
1 g fiber
10 g protein

This fish has added omega-6 oils, caramel color, and STPP. Same with the Gorton's Beer-Battered Fish Fillets

Signature Grilled Tilapia Fish Fillets

80 calories
2 g fat
140 mg sodium
15 g protein

This omega-6-heavy fish contains the controversial additive propyl gallate, which is banned in other countries as an endocrine disruptor

SNOWS BUMBLE BEE

Minced Canned Clams

25 calories
0 fat
350 mg sodium
25 g carbs
0 fiber
3 g protein

Contain STPP and EDTA

MACKNIGHT

Atlantic Salmon Burgers

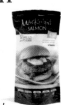

160 calories
7 g fat
245 mg sodium
0 g fiber
22 g protein

Farm-raised salmon!

PHILLIPS

Maryland Style Crab Cakes

160 calories
10 g fat
500 mg sodium
0 g fiber
11 g protein

Contains the additive disodium EDTA

HANDY

Crab Cakes

160 calories
11 g fat
2 g sat fat
440 mg sodium
10 g protein

Sugar in the ingredient list 4 times

DUCKTRAP

Smoked Atlantic Salmon

130 calories
9 g fat
690 mg sodium
0 fiber
11 g protein

FRENCH FRIES

When it comes to French fries, in the immortal words of Frankie Valli, "Grease is the word." What happens when the fry hits your tastebuds—not to mention what happens when it hits your bloodstream—is all about the quality of the oil it's fried in. And back in 2006, many of the fast-food restaurants made a big deal about changing recipes in order to avoid using those dangerous partially hydrogenated oils that contain trans fats.

Trans fats increase heart disease risk by lowering HDL cholesterol (the good cholesterol) and raising LDL cholesterol (the bad cholesterol). More closely related to plastic than to any natural food substance, trans fats act like flypaper on the insides of your arteries, gumming up the works and increasing your risk of blockage. So naturally, the world applauded when all the big chain restaurants eliminated trans fats from their menus and everyone happily went back to eating their fried foods, this time guilt-free. But that is not the end of the story.

The American Heart Association recommends that no more than 1 percent of your total daily calorie intake be from trans fats;

While most fast food restaurants have at least reduced the trans fats in their fries, a 4-oz. order of Long John Silver's French Fries still has a whopping 3 grams of trans fats. The source of all that trans fat is the partially hydro-genated vege-table shortening they're cooked with.

WORST FRENCH FRIES

Long John Silver's French Fries

300 calories
15 g fat
3 g trans fat
430 mg sodium
0 g sugar
4 g protein

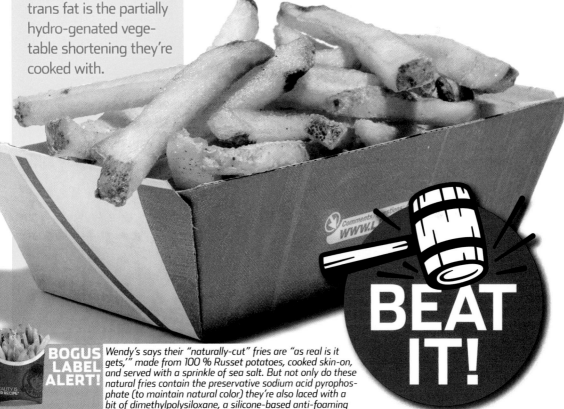

BOGUS LABEL ALERT!

Wendy's says their "naturally-cut" fries are "as real is it gets,'" made from 100 % Russet potatoes, cooked skin-on, and served with a sprinkle of sea salt. But not only do these natural fries contain the preservative sodium acid pyrophosphate (to maintain natural color) they're also laced with a bit of dimethylpolysiloxane, a silicone-based anti-foaming agent that is also an ingredient in Silly Putty.

BEAT IT!

for the average American, that translates to about 1.5 to 2 grams per day. But oops: Under FDA rules, it's legal for companies to say their food is "trans fat free" even if they contain up to 0.5 g of trans fat per serving. Which is how places like White Castle can get away with saying "0 grams of trans fats per serving" even when trans fats are still lurking in the ingredients list of their French fries and other foods. In fact, you can easily exceed your total daily limit of trans fats in one sitting at a fast food joint, while eating only food that's labeled "trans fat free."

Can you believe they get away with that? Here's how to fight back.

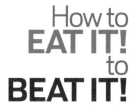

How to
EAT IT!
to
BEAT IT!

The French may lay claim to the fry, but potatoes are an all-American food, originally discovered and brought to Europe by Spanish explorers from the New World in the 1500s. And the process by which a tuber turns into something Ronald McDonald can sell is a miracle of American ingenuity.

Your humble tater is yanked from the ground and placed into a truck with, oh, between 25 and 30 tons of other potatoes. Then it's shipped to a processing plant, where it's graded for quality, steam peeled, barrel washed, trimmed of blemishes, and then dropped into a water pump that shoots it at 70 miles an hour through a grid made of knives to create the signature shoestring. Then these shoestrings are processed, first by blanching, which removes the natural sugars and sets up the internal texture of the French fry, making it fluffy like a baked potato. Then they are dried and fried, which sets up the crisp outer texture, and then sent quickly through a freeze tunnel, which brings their temperature to under 10 degrees so they can be shipped all over the world.

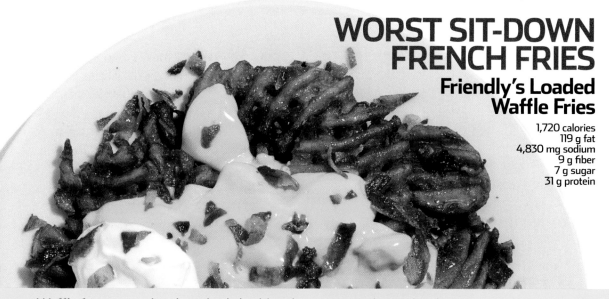

WORST SIT-DOWN FRENCH FRIES

Friendly's Loaded Waffle Fries

1,720 calories
119 g fat
4,830 mg sodium
9 g fiber
7 g sugar
31 g protein

Waffle fries topped with melted cheddar cheese sauce, bacon, and sour cream, served with ranch dressing on the side. It's no wonder that 1,070 of the 1,720 calories are fat calories!

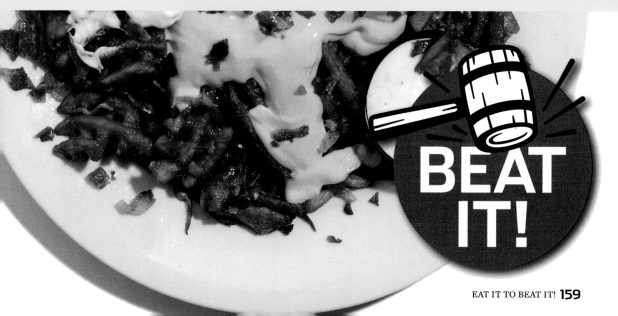

BEAT IT!

THE FRENCH FRY RULES

KNOW YOUR OILS. If there are partially hydrogenated oils in the ingredient list, those fries contain some trans fats. Partially hydrogenated oils are liquid oils that have been hydrogenated to make them more solid. The more solid the oil, the higher the smoke point, the better for high-heat cooking. Forcing hydrogen into liquid oils changes the chemical structure so they become more solid. Partially hydrogenating the oils leaves them a little soft, which makes them more manageable for cooking, but also creates the trans fats that are so dangerous. Fully hydrogenated oils do not contain trans fats.

GO FILTER FREE. Most restaurants use an oil-filtration system to increase the lifespan of their fry oil. That means they pour in a fine powder, like diatomaceous earth or synthetic magnesium sulfate, to soak up the impurities and then run the oil through a micro-filter to take out the impurities. This also turns once "healthy" oils into highly refined oils devoid of their nutrient content. Ask the manager at the restaurant if they filter their oil or if they replace it daily.

KEEP IT YELLOW. Darker fries are a sign of high levels of the cancer-causing chemical acrylamide, which occurs naturally during the frying process. But shorter frying times, lower temperatures, cleaner oil, and freezing the fries before cooking helps to lower their acrylamide content. Look for fries that are golden yellow, not tan, brown, or burnt. The longer the frying time, and the older the fry oil, the more acrylamide and the darker the fry.

TROUBLESHOOT YOUR FRIES

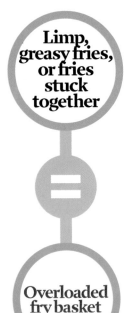

Limp, greasy fries, or fries stuck together

=

Overloaded fry basket

BEWARE THE BUDGET FRY. Restaurants often buy "budget fries," which cost them less but are shorter and contain less potato solids. If you're served a plate of fries that are all about 2 inches long, you're eating budget fries, which are processed to contain more water and less potato.

THE FRENCH FRY ADVANTAGE

Lower Blood Pressure

A USDA study of potatoes recently found levels of phytochemicals such as flavonoids and kukoamines that rival the amounts found in broccoli, spinach, and Brussels sprouts. Kukoamines, previously thought to reside only in the Chinese medicinal plant *Lycium chinense,* have been shown to lower blood pressure by decreasing free-radical damage and inflammation. Now, I'm not saying that eating French fries will lower your blood pressure (there is all that salt to consider), but the potato has gotten a bad rap as just an empty starch. There's more to taters than meets the eye, and as an occasional indulgence there are worse snacks out there.

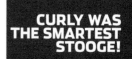

CURLY WAS THE SMARTEST STOOGE!

A recent study from researchers at the Psycho-metrics Centre of the University of Cambridge found that "liking" curly fries on Facebook was one of the best predictors of high intelligence. Other predictors? Liking thunderstorms, the Colbert Report, and science. Although I don't think eating a large portion of Arby's 630-calorie curly fries is all that smart.

BEST SIT-DOWN FRIES

Longhorn Steakhouse Seasoned Fries

Longhorn Steakhouse serves up a plate of crispy French fries for only 280 calories and 135 mg of sodium. Lightly seasoned and hold the guilt!

280 calories
13 g fat
135 mg sodium

EAT IT!

BEST FAST-FOOD FRIES

520 calories
26 g fat
135 mg sodium

Elevation Burger Fries

Elevation Burger fries are some of the only fast-food fries that are just potatoes, salt, and oil. To cook their fries, they use Bertolli classic olive oil, which has a higher smoke point than extra virgin olive oil. And these fries don't contain any hydrogenated oils, anti-foaming agents, or color preservers like most fast-food fries do. One boat of fries is 520 calories, though, so split the boat and enjoy some French fries that are as close to a natural, whole food, fast-food fry as you're going to get.

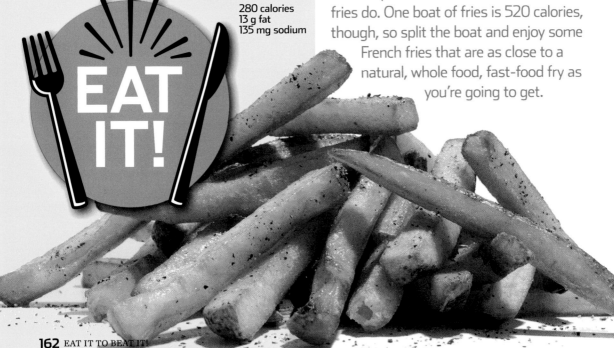

OTHER GOOD FAST-FOOD FRENCH FRIES:

SONIC
French Fries (small)
- 220 calories
- 10 g of fat
- 220 mg sodium

MCDONALD'S
French Fries (small)
- 230 calories
- 11 g fat
- 160 mg sodium

WENDY'S
French Fries (value)
- 220 calories
- 11 g fat
- 240 mg sodium

BURGER KING
French Fries (value size)
- 240 calories
- 10 g fat
- 330 mg sodium

CHICK-FIL-A
Waffle Potato Fries (small)
- 310 calories
- 16g fat
- 140 mg sodium

WHITE CASTLE
French Fries (small)
- 330 calories
- 21 g fat
- 50 mg sodium

OTHER GOOD SIT-DOWN FRIES:

TGI FRIDAY'S
Seasoned Fries
- 270 calories
- 22 g fat
- 980 mg sodium

RED LOBSTER
French Fries
- 330 calories
- 17 g fat
- 740 mg sodium

IHOP
Seasoned Fries (not the appetizer, the side)
- 300 calories
- 12 g fat
- 490 mg sodium

HARD ROCK CAFE
Seasoned French Fries
- 287 calories
- N/A fat
- N/A sodium

WORST FAST-FOOD FRIES:

WENDY'S
Chili Cheese Fries
- 530 calories
- 28 g fat
- 1,050 mg sodium

POPEYES
Cajun Fries
- 770 calories
- 3.5 g trans fat
- 1,700 mg of sodium

JACK IN THE BOX
Bacon Cheddar Potato Wedges
- 679 calories
- 41 g fat
- 1,251 mg sodium

FIVE GUYS
Fries (large)
- 1,314 calories
- 57 g of fat
- 1,327 g sodium

ARBY'S
Curly Fries (large)
- 630 calories
- 35 g fat
- 1,420 mg sodium

BEAT IT!

WORST SIT-DOWN FRIES:

OUTBACK AUSSIE
Cheese Fries (small)
- 1,218 calories
- 91 g fat
- 1,783 mg sodium

CHILI'S
Texas Cheese Fries
- 1,730 calories
- 117 g fat
- 5,280 mg sodium

CHEESECAKE FACTORY
Plain French Fries
- 690 calories
- 13 g sat fat
- 450 mg sodium

NATHAN'S FAMOUS
Chili Cheese Fries
- 1,070 calories
- 72 g fat
- 1,010 mg sodium

HOT BREAKFAST

By now, you've probably read enough about nutrition to know that skipping breakfast is right up there with smoking, texting while driving, and swimming with orcas while wearing a seal costume on the list of Really Bad Health Ideas. In fact, with so much hype about the importance of breakfast, it's not unreasonable to think that cracking open a vending machine and Hoovering out its contents for breakfast is preferable to just skipping the meal entirely.

But take my word for it, there are breakfasts worth skipping. Your best bet is always to prepare something yourself—take a few extra minutes in the morning to crack a couple of eggs and toss an English muffin into the toaster. But if you can't, then tread carefully into the world of breakfast. The road to hell is paved with sausage patties.

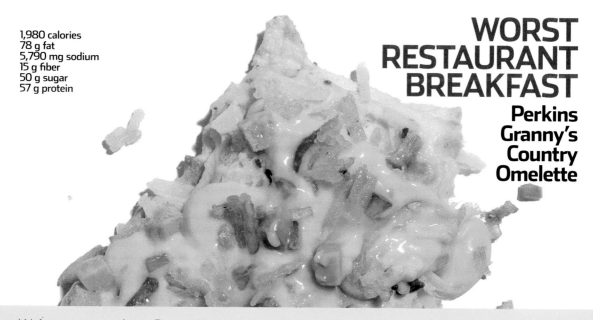

1,980 calories
78 g fat
5,790 mg sodium
15 g fiber
50 g sugar
57 g protein

WORST RESTAURANT BREAKFAST

Perkins Granny's Country Omelette

We're not sure where Granny's country is, but we think she may have spent her formative years in Fatslavia. With a day's worth of calories and three days' worth of sodium, it may be time to revoke Granny's visa.

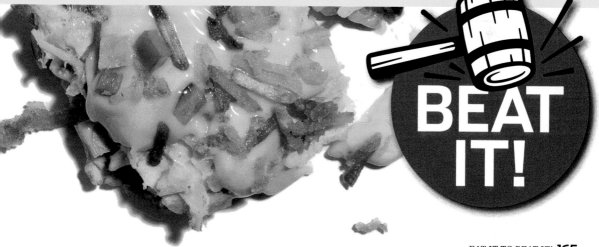

BEAT IT!

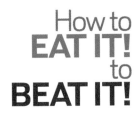 How to **EAT IT!** to **BEAT IT!**

Even if it's just a glass of milk and a spoonful of peanut butter, having something to jumpstart your morning—especially if it contains protein and fiber—will help you eat less during the rest of the day. One study found that men who ate 3 scrambled eggs for breakfast consumed 400 fewer calories throughout the day compared to when they ate a bagel breakfast of similar calories. Four hundred fewer calories a day means you'd lose nearly 42 pounds in a year!

THE BREAKFAST RULES

SKIP THE FREEZER SECTION. Try as I might, I can't find any pre-packaged hot breakfast that doesn't have trans fats, processed cheese, artificial colorings, or mechanically separated meat products. If you're eating at home, make it yourself.

CHOOSE QUALITY CARBS. Make sure you add some fruit, vegetables, or whole grains to your morning meal.

BACON & EGGHEADS

Kids who eat breakfast every day have significantly higher IQ scores, according to researchers from the University of Pennsylvania. They examined 1,269 children and found that those who did not eat breakfast regularly had IQ scores that were 4.6 points lower than children who always ate breakfast.

THE BREAKFAST ADVANTAGE

Lose Weight

A recent study published in the *American Journal of Clinical Nutrition* found that people who ate 350 calories of eggs and lean beef for breakfast consumed 290 fewer calories throughout the day than those who ate 350 calories of cereal. There was also a 30 percent reduction in the desire to eat and a 20 percent reduction in the production of the hunger hormone ghrelin.

Lower Cholesterol

A recent study of 26,902 men, published in the journal *Circulation,* found that those who skipped breakfast had a 27 percent higher risk of heart attack or death from coronary heart disease.

HOW TO LOSE YOUR LUNCH BEFORE BREAKFAST

If you like sausage, don't look too closely at the label. The best sausage patties will be made of pork and flavorings, but there are some that contain a bit of "Mechanically Separated Turkey." This is a paste-like substance derived from the leftover turkey carcass that can contain skeletal meat, skin, and up to 1 percent bone fragment. You'll find this delicacy in Special K Flatbread Sausage Egg and Cheese Breakfast Sandwiches, Weight Watchers Smart Ones Breakfasts entrees with sausage, and others.

BEST HOT RESTAURANT BREAKFAST

Panera Bread Breakfast Power on Whole Grain

340 calories
15 g fat
920 mg sodium
4 g fiber
3 g sugar
16 g protein

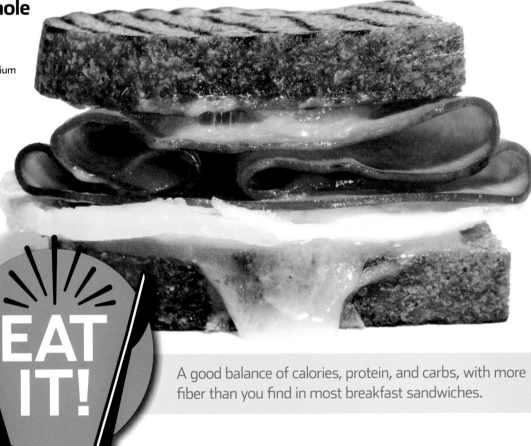

EAT IT!

A good balance of calories, protein, and carbs, with more fiber than you find in most breakfast sandwiches.

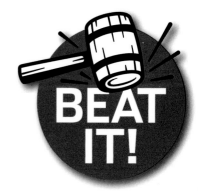

CARL'S JR.
Bacon, Egg & Cheese Biscuit

480 calories
30 g fat
1,180 mg sodium
3 g fiber
3 g sugar
15 g protein

BLIMPIE
Bluffin Bacon Egg & Cheese

320 calories
16 g fat
1,090 mg sodium
2 g fiber
2 g sugar
17 g protein

AU BON PAIN
Ham and Cheese Croissant

410 calories
22 g fat
700 mg sodium
1 g fiber
6 g sugar
18 g protein

Egg, Bacon, Cheddar on Ciabatta

470 calories
22 g fat
1,050 mg sodium
2 g fiber
2 g sugar
28 g protein

SUBWAY
Bacon, Egg and Cheese on 3" Flatbread

210 calories
9 g fat
560 mg sodium
1 g fiber
2 g sugar
11 g protein

BURGER KING
Sausage Breakfast Burrito

290 calories
17 g fat
830 mg sodium
1 g fiber
2 g sugar
14 g protein

TIM HORTON
Bacon Egg and Cheese Wrap

270 calories
16 g fat
630 mg sodium
2 g fiber
1 g sugar
13 g protein

CHEESECAKE FACTORY
French Toast with bacon

1,849 calories
65 g sat fat
3,114 mg sodium
98 g carbs

Monte Cristo, Classic Style

1,966 calories
54 g sat fat
2,872 mg sodium
161 g carbs

BURGER KING
Ultimate Breakfast Platter

1,450 calories
84 g fat
2,920 mg sodium
5 g fiber
41 g sugar
40 g protein

DENNY'S
Grand Slamwich with hash browns

1,530 calories
102 g fat
3,690 mg sodium
5 g fiber
52 g protein
11 g sugar

STEAK 'N SHAKE
Steakburger Slinger Skillet— Sausage

1,650 calories
136 g fat
2,700 mg sodium
8 g fiber
2 g sugar
61 g protein

IHOP
Country Chicken Fried Steak and Eggs with sausage gravy

1,850 calories
115 g fat
4,550 mg sodium
8 g fiber
12 g sugar
61 g protein

ICE CREAM

BOGUS LABEL ALERT!

"Frozen Dairy Dessert." You would assume that's the definition of ice cream, but in fact, the word *"dairy"* basically means "there's not much dairy." The FDA says that to be labeled ice cream, a dessert must be at least 10 percent milk fat. While it might sound appealing to have less fat in your ice cream, manufacturers will simply replace those dairy fats with other fats like palm oil, soybean oil, and even partially hydrogenated oils (i.e., trans fats).

In the *Mad Men* days, the height of fame in America was to have a sandwich named after you at the famous Carnegie Deli. But nowadays, we celebrate icons like Stephen Colbert and Jerry Garcia by naming ice cream flavors after them. Sadly, I think this chapter is going to ruin my chances of ever enjoying a scoop of Baskin-Robbins "Zincky Dink Chocolate Chunk."

At its core, ice cream should just be milk, sugar, cream, and maybe a little fruit. But ice cream, especially when it gets sidetracked into shakes, sundaes, and other frozen diversions, is among the most corrupted foods on the planet. If Elliot Ness were alive today, he'd be giving bank robbers a free pass and going after Baskin-Robbins instead. Among the common additives in ice cream today (and in the immortal words of Dave Barry, "I am not making this up"): antifreeze, wood pulp, and the anal scent glands of beavers (called "castoreum," it's among the "natural flavors" found in some vanilla- or raspberry-flavored desserts). Here's the scoop.

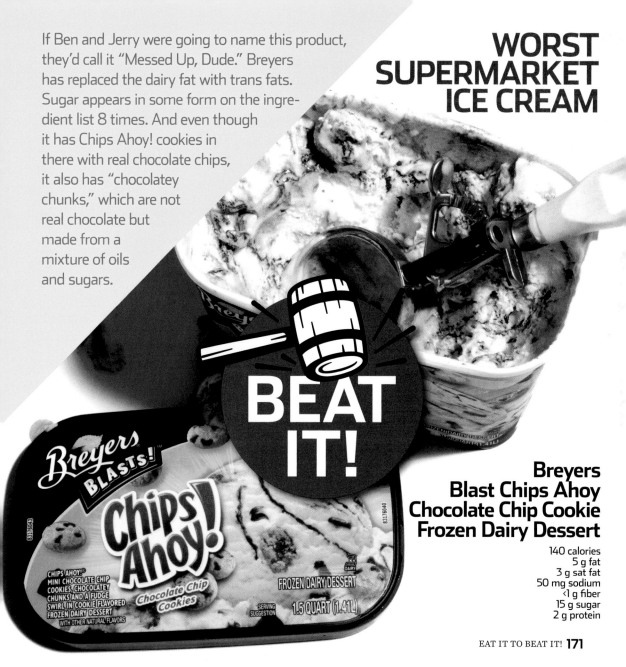

If Ben and Jerry were going to name this product, they'd call it "Messed Up, Dude." Breyers has replaced the dairy fat with trans fats. Sugar appears in some form on the ingredient list 8 times. And even though it has Chips Ahoy! cookies in there with real chocolate chips, it also has "chocolatey chunks," which are not real chocolate but made from a mixture of oils and sugars.

WORST SUPERMARKET ICE CREAM

BEAT IT!

Breyers Blast Chips Ahoy Chocolate Chip Cookie Frozen Dairy Dessert

140 calories
5 g fat
3 g sat fat
50 mg sodium
<1 g fiber
15 g sugar
2 g protein

Breyers BLASTS!
Chips Ahoy!
Chocolate Chip Cookies

CHIPS AHOY! MINI CHOCOLATE CHIP COOKIES, CHOCOLATEY CHUNKS AND A FUDGE SWIRL IN COOKIE FLAVORED FROZEN DAIRY DESSERT WITH OTHER NATURAL FLAVORS

FROZEN DAIRY DESSERT

SERVING SUGGESTION 1.5 QUART (1.41L)

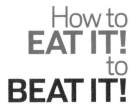

How to
EAT IT!
to
BEAT IT!

People—and by that I mean, really, really rich people with armies of servants—have been enjoying ice cream since the first century A.D. But it became available to the likes of you and me only 150 years ago, when modern refrigeration methods were invented. And once that happened, really, really rich people with armies of servants—and by that I mean major food manufacturers—quickly figured out a way to make this simple indulgence really, really complicated.

THE ICE CREAM RULES

DON'T STRESS ON FAT. Ice cream is a high-calorie treat with lots of fat. The closer you get to pure ice cream, the more calories from fat you're going to have. Häagen-Dazs Vanilla is about the purest ice cream on the market. It has 5 ingredients and doesn't use any gums. It has 250 calories, 17 g fat, 10 g sat fat, 50 g sodium, 0 fiber, 19 g sugar, and 4 g protein. But it's when ice cream makers start upping the sugar content with additives that ice cream really gets bad for you.

SIMPLIFY. Traditionally, ice cream is just a frozen mixture of cream, milk, sugar, and sometimes eggs. Commercial ice cream manufacturers almost always use emulsifiers like guar gum, xantham gum, vegetable oil, corn extracts, and more. The more of these you're getting, the less actual real ice cream you're getting.

TOP WISELY. Fruity and chocolaty ice cream flavors come with a lot of baggage, and mostly it's not actual fruit or chocolate. Strawberry and chocolate chip are two of the most popular ice

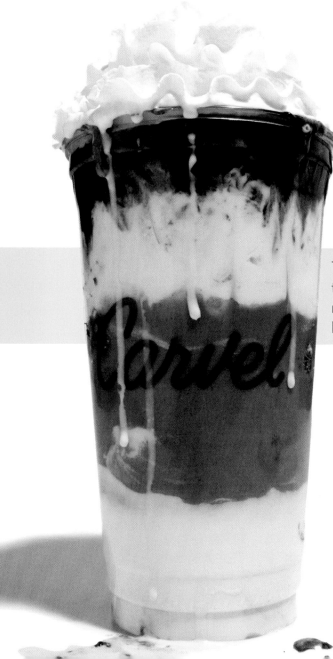

WORST RESTAURANT ICE CREAM

Carvel Peanut Butter Cup Sundae Dasher Large

1,960 calories
111 g fat
1,270 mg sodium
14 g fiber
139 g sugar
41 g protein

There are a lot of Carvel offerings that top the 1,000-calorie mark and more than a few that are over 1,500. But this one takes the calorie cake.

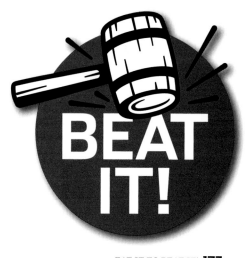

BEAT IT!

cream flavors but a lot of the time you're just getting vegetable oil mixed with flavoring and sweetener instead of the real thing. At home, you're always best off having a simple ice cream and adding your own fruit, nuts, and dark chocolate.

GET SMALL. When ordering out, choose the small or even the kiddie size. Every half-cup you shovel into the bowl is another 200 to 300 calories. And savor every bite: a study published in the *Journal of Clinical Endocrinology and Metabolism* in 2010 measured satiety in patients who ate a helping of ice cream in five minutes versus 30 minutes, and found that those who ate slower had much higher levels of the appetite regulating hormone PYY after the meal.

From the Files of Dr. Softee, MD

Diagnosis: **Sphenopalantine Ganglioneuralgia**
Also known as: **Ice Cream Headache**
Symptoms: **Patient presented with crushing cranial pain shortly after first bites of vanilla chocolate swirl.**

Pathology:

Cold ice cream changes the temperature in the back of a patient's throat, right at the convergence of the internal carotid artery, which feeds the brain blood and the anterior cerebral artery, which is the start of patient's brain tissue. When the cold hits quickly, it causes these two arteries to dilate and contract, and the brain reads these movements through tiny receptors on the outer brain wall called meninges, causing a rapid onset headache.

Solution:

Patient was advised to place her tongue on the roof of her mouth to warm it up, or to drink something room temperature. And to take it easy next time.

GO LEFT. Here's a trick for cutting down on dessert calories: If you're right-handed, hold the spoon in your left hand, and eat dessert that way (and vice versa). It will naturally reduce the number of calories you eat.

AVOID ANTIFREEZE. There's an ingredient hiding in some ice creams that might give you serious pause. It's antifreeze, otherwise known as propylene glycol. Skinny Cow, Breyers Fat-free, and Carb Smart, among other brands, use it in their "light" ice creams to make them easier to scoop when you open the container.

An Easy Alternative to Ice Cream

Frozen Banana Whips

What You Do

Slice up bananas and freeze them. Toss a half cup of frozen banana slices in a blender and blend until smooth. Add a teaspoon or two of honey.

Get Creative

Make your own flavors by adding 2 or 3 tablespoons of chocolate spread, peanut butter, or berries. Add a splash of cream or yogurt to make it creamier.

BEST SUPERMARKET ICE CREAM

Häagen-Dazs Vanilla Ice Cream

250 calories
17 g fat
10 g sat fat
50 g sodium
0 fiber
19 g sugar
4 g protein

A high-calorie indulgence, but this is about the purest ice cream on the market. It has 5 ingredients and doesn't use any gums.

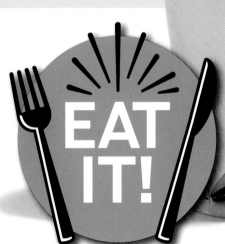

EAT IT!

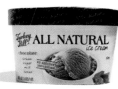

TURKEY HILL
Ice Cream, Chocolate All Natural

170 calories
10 g fat
6 g sat fat
35 mg sodium
1 g fiber
17 g sugar
3 g protein

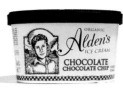

ALDEN'S ORGANIC
Ice Cream, Chocolate Chocolate Chip

180 calories
11 g fat
7 g sat fat
35 mg sodium
1 g fiber
15 g sugar
3 g protein

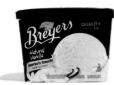

BREYERS
Natural Vanilla Ice Cream

130 calories
7 g fat
4 g sat fat
35 mg sodium
0 g fiber
14 g sugar
3 g protein

*Breyers All Natural line
is notably low in calories
and wacky additives*

WEGMANS
Food You Feel Good About Organic Vanilla Premium Ice Cream

270 calories
18 g fat
11 g sat fat
70 mg sodium
0 g fiber
21 g sugar
5 g protein

BREYERS
Chocolate Chip

140 calories
5 g fat
4 g sat fat
35 mg sodium
0 fiber
16 g sugar
2 g protein

*It's a frozen dairy desert with
"chocolate flavored chips"*

BEN & JERRY'S
Chubby Hubby

340 calories
21 g fat
150 mg sodium
2 g fiber
25 g sugar
7 g protein

*High calorie, plus contains
palm kernel oil and corn oil*

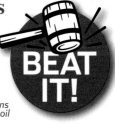

SKINNY COW
Ice Cream Caramel Cone Low Fat Single Serve

160 calories
2.5 g fat
2 g sat fat
85 mg sodium
4 g fiber
21 g sugar
4 g protein

*A faux health food! "Chocolatey dipped
waffle cone" (not real chocolate), antifreeze
(propylene glycol), wood pulp (microcrystalline cellulose), and seaweed (carrageenan)*

EDY'S
Slow Churned Ice Cream, Butter Pecan No Sugar Added Light

120 calories
5 g fat
2 g sat fat
80 mg sodium
2 g fiber
3 g sugar
3 g protein

*If you're wondering what exactly is going to get "slow churned,"
there are 3 asterisks in the ingredient list pointing out the
possible laxative side effects of these ingredients: maltitol syrup,
polydextrose, and sorbitol.*

BEST RESTAURANT ICE CREAM

Dairy Queen
Small Caramel Sundae

300 calories
7 g fat
150 mg sodium
0 g fiber
36 g sugar
6 g protein

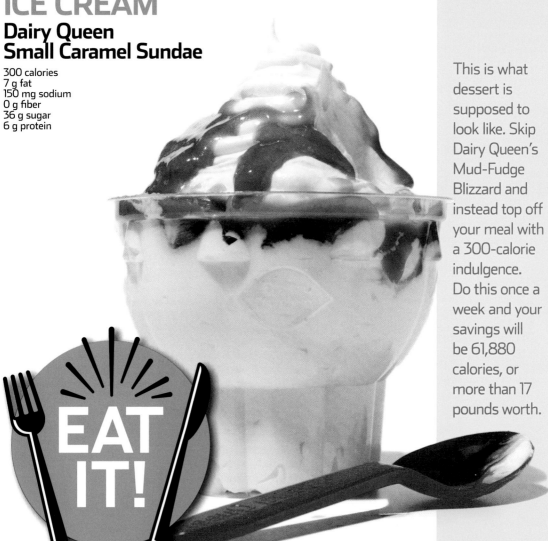

This is what dessert is supposed to look like. Skip Dairy Queen's Mud-Fudge Blizzard and instead top off your meal with a 300-calorie indulgence. Do this once a week and your savings will be 61,880 calories, or more than 17 pounds worth.

EAT IT!

STEAK 'N SHAKE

Chocolate Milk Shake (kids)

390 calories
12 g fat
220 mg sodium
1 g fiber
57 g sugar
11 g protein

BASKIN-ROBBINS

Ice Cream Float (mini)

240 calories
10 g fat
85 mg sodium
0 fiber
38 g sugar
3 g protein

COLD STONE CREAMERY

Berry Berry Berry Good ("Like it" size)

360 calories
20 g fat
90 mg sodium
2 g fiber
37 g sugar
5 g protein

FRIENDLY'S

Reese's Peanut Butter Cup 5 Scoop

1,190 calories
70 g fat
460 mg sodium
7 g fiber
86 g sugar
21 g protein

A&W

Chocolate Fudge Blendrrr 32-oz

1,010 calories
59 g fat
220 mg sodium
97 g sugar
8 g protein

APPLEBEE'S

Chocolate Chip Cookie Sundae

1,590 calories
75 g fat
47 g sat fat
990 mg sodium
8 g fiber
18 g protein

DAIRY QUEEN

Georgia Mud Fudge Blizzard (large)

1,190 calories
62 g fat
740 mg sodium
8 g fiber
114 g sugar
22 g protein

FRIENDLY'S

Hunka Chunka Pb Fudge Lava Cake Sundae

1,770 calories
107 g fat
36 g fat
1,050 mg sodium
15 g fiber
112 g sugar
37 g protein

DENNY'S

Oreo Milk Shake

1,440 calories
73 g fat
36 g sat fat
750 mg sodium
3 g fiber
25 g protein
123 g sugar

JACK-IN-THE-BOX

Oreo Cookie with Whipped Topping 24 oz

1,170 calories
61 g fat
560 mg sodium
2 g fiber
105 g sugar
19 g protein

STEAK 'N SHAKE

Nutter Butter Milk Shake (large)

1,650 calories
73 g fat
1,360 mg sodium
2 g fiber
184 g sugar
35 g protein

BASKIN-ROBBINS

Chocolate Chip Cookie Dough Shake (large)

1,600 calories
72 g fat
740 mg sodium
2 fiber
181 g sugar
30 g protein

SONIC

Large Chocolate Shake

1,410 calories
58 g fat
720 mg sodium
0 fiber
107 g sugar
16 g protein

COLD STONE CREAMERY

Cake n Shake

1,320 calories
69 g fat
910 mg sodium
2 g fiber
133 g sugar
19 g protein

BEAT IT!

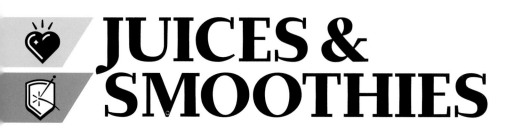

JUICES & SMOOTHIES

Juice, you really let us down. Once, we looked up to you as a hero, a star, a national treasure. Then one day we're watching TV, and a white Ford Bronco is racing down the highway, and . . .

Oh, wait, different juice.

But not really. Like the football star turned serial convict, the other kind of juice has turned out to be a lot nastier in real life than its public image would let on. From cranberry cocktail to fruit punch, juice—and its Kato Kaelin–like sidekick, the smoothie—needs to be eyed with a little more suspicion than we once thought.

The problem: added sugar. While fruit on its own has plenty of sugar already—as anyone who's ever bitten into a ripe summer peach can attest—food marketers just aren't happy unless they've taken something healthy and natural and made it weird and, often, unhealthy. Sorry, juice makers: The glove fits, and we cannot acquit.

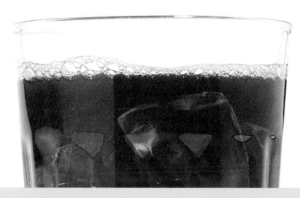

WORST JUICE

IHOP
Cranberry Juice

210 calories
0 fat
65 mg sodium
3 g fiber
53 g sugar
0 protein

Somehow this IHOP beverage packs 53 g of sugar in one glass of juice—that's the equivalent of two whole Snickers bars! "IHOP" describes what your kids will be doing for the next hour after downing this "healthy" beverage.

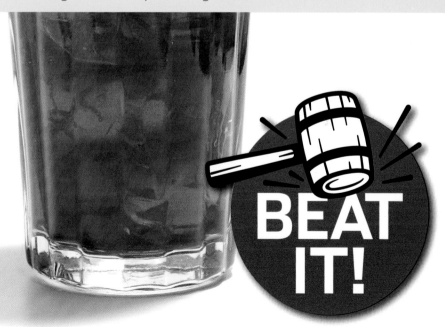

BEAT IT!

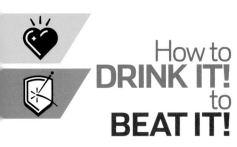

How to DRINK IT! to BEAT IT!

Even the best juices in the world aren't as good as eating real, fresh fruit. That's because fruit is naturally high in sugar and calories—which is fine when you're eating, say, an orange or a peach. But not fine when you're drinking the equivalent of a half dozen of them, which is what you're often getting with a large glass of fruit juice. More important, juice has most of the fiber squeezed out of it, so juice just isn't as nutritious as the original fruit it came from. So even if you squeeze it yourself, juice is a compromise. A delicious compromise, but a compromise just the same. And that's before food companies start working their mischief.

THE JUICE RULES

GIVE IT 100 PERCENT. "Made from real fruit" doesn't mean anything, other than that at some point at least one slice of fruit came in contact with this concoction. You want to choose juices that are 100 percent fruit juice. Make sure the ingredients list juices, and no added sugars.

DON'T FALL IN THE "DRINK." Fruit "drink" is not juice. It's sugar water and food coloring. In many cases, there is little or no nutritional value to fruit drink. Same is true for "fruit-flavored beverages."

COCKTAILS ARE FOR GROWN-UPS. Fruit juice cocktails are often just a mixture of water, juice concentrates, and sugar. Same with fruit juice blends. These concoctions might be only 15 percent fruit juice.

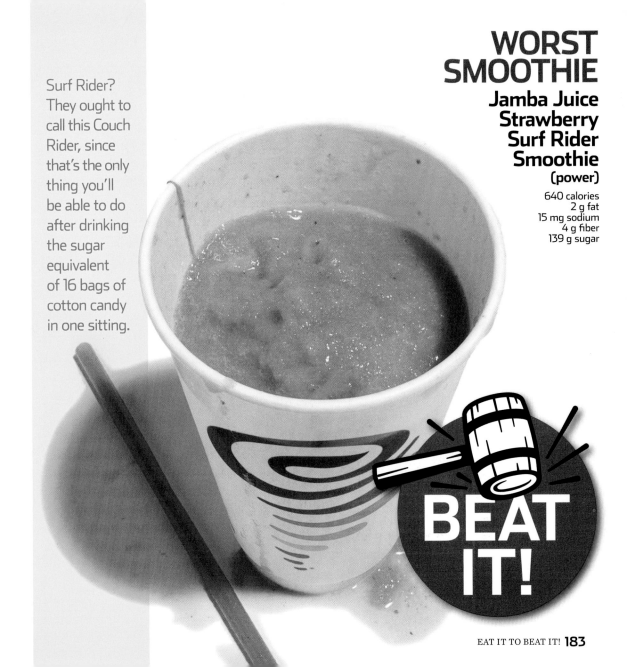

Surf Rider? They ought to call this Couch Rider, since that's the only thing you'll be able to do after drinking the sugar equivalent of 16 bags of cotton candy in one sitting.

WORST SMOOTHIE

Jamba Juice Strawberry Surf Rider Smoothie
(power)

640 calories
2 g fat
15 mg sodium
4 g fiber
139 g sugar

BEAT IT!

AVOID "DIET" AND "LIGHT." Usually these words mean one thing: sucralose. This artificial sweetener has been shown to spike blood sugar just as much as natural sugars.

BEWARE OF SERVING SIZE TRICKERY. Most "individual" bottles of juice hide their true calorie and sugar load by increasing the serving size in the bottle. Most Naked Juices, for example, are labeled as two servings, even though you'll of course drink the whole bottle. So the 30 grams of sugar you see on the back is actually 60 grams if you drink the whole thing!

WATER IT DOWN. A great way to get all the vitamins and flavor you want from juice without the ridiculous calorie count is to add juice to sparking water. Put on your sunglasses, turn on *Absolutely Fabulous,* and pretend you're having a mimosa.

A KICK IN THE ARSENIC

Researchers recently found that people who regularly drink apple juice have on average 19 percent higher levels of arsenic in their urine than those who do not; grape juice drinkers have 20 percent higher levels. They recommend limiting yourself to no more than 8 to 12 ounces a day (4 to 6 ounces for kids up to 6). The FDA recently set a standard of no more than 10 ppb (parts per billion) of arsenic in juice, but a study by Consumer Reports *found that many commercial juices reached or exceeded that level.*

 APPLE JUICE: Apple & Eve, Great Value (Walmart), and Mott's: some samples had more than 10 ppb.

 GRAPE JUICE: Walgreens and Welch's: some samples had more than 10 ppb.

THE JUICE ADVANTAGE

Boost Immunity

Orange juice is a no-nonsense dose of Vitamin C, important for many bodily processes including wound-healing and maintaining cartilage. A 2006 study noted that Vitamin C improves components of the immune system such as antimicrobial and natural killer cell activities, and multiple studies show that adequate intake of Vitamin C is helpful for shortening and lessening the symptoms of colds.

Grape juice (another American favorite) has also been linked to immunity. A study published in the *Journal of Medicinal Food* in 2011 found that 100 percent grape juice increased T-cell activity (the cells that seek out and destroy invaders).

Lower Cholesterol

A 2010 study from the journal *Nutrition Research* linked OJ to lower cholesterol. Participants who already had high cholesterol who drank a daily glass of OJ from concentrate had lower cholesterol, and both the normal and high cholesterol groups had higher rates of transfer of free cholesterol to HDL. "Low-energy" cranberry juice has also been linked to lower LDL cholesterol, according to a 2011 study published in *Nutrition Research*.

BEST SUPERMARKET JUICE

Lakewood Organic 100% Fruit Juice, Pure Cranberry

75 calories
0 fat
5 mg sodium
1 g fiber
7 g sugar
1 g protein

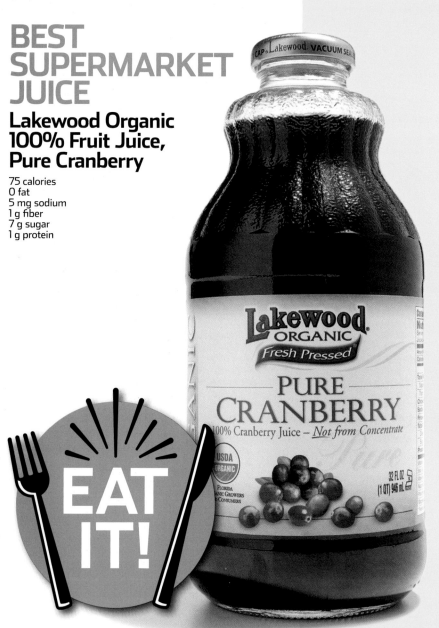

EAT IT!

The ingredients: fresh pressed juice from certified organic cranberries. And that's it. No additives, fillers, extra sugars, unnecessary vitamins, or weird preservatives. Just the juice of some healthy fruit.

ODWALLA
Carrot Juice

100 calories
0 fat
240 mg sodium
1 g fiber
19 g sugar
3 g protein

Just juice, no added sugar (nutrition facts based on whole bottle as 1 serving)

R.W. KNUDSEN
Just Black Current Juice

100 calories
0 fat
5 mg sodium
15 g sugar
1 g protein

JUICY JUICE
Fruit Punch

120 calories
0 fat
20 mg sodium
26 g sugar
0 protein

100 percent juice, no added sugars

UNCLE MATT'S
Orange Juice with pulp

110 calories
0 fat
0 sodium
22 g sugar
2 g protein

V8
Original Low Sodium

50 calories
0 fat
140 mg sodium
2 g fiber
7 g sugar
2 g protein

SMOOTHIES:

NAKED
Green Machine

140 calories
0 g fat
15 mg sodium
0 g fiber
28 g sugar
2 g protein

LIFEWAY
Lowfat Blueberry Kefir

140 calories
2 g fat
125 mg sodium
20 g sugar
11 g protein

BOLTHOUSE FARMS
Strawberry Banana

130 calories
0 fat
15 mg sodium
2 g fiber
22 g sugar
1 g protein

BEST RESTAURANT JUICE

Jamba Juice Carrot Juice

100 calories
0 fat
170 mg sodium
0 fiber
20 g sugar
3 g protein

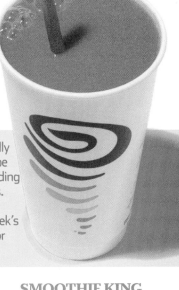

Carrots are so naturally sweet that they can be squeezed without adding any additional sugars. The 12-ounce Jamba Juice has a whole week's worth of vitamin A for just 100 calories.

DENNY'S
Orange Grove Smoothie

120 calories
0 fat
30 mg sodium
0 fiber
22 g sugar
1 g protein

STARBUCKS
Orange Mango Smoothie

270 calories
1.5 g fat
0 mg sodium
6 g fiber
37 g sugar
16 g protein

SMOOTHIE KING
Pure Recharge Mango Strawberry Energy

210 calories
0 fat
120 mg sodium
2 g fiber
50 g sugar
0 protein

COLD STONE CREAMERY
Berry Trinity

160 calories
1.5 g fat
35 mg sodium
8 g fiber
21 g sugar
2 g protein

WORST SUPERMARKET JUICE

Ocean Spray Diet Cran-Grape Juice Drink

5 calories
0 fat
50 mg sodium
2 g sugar
0 protein

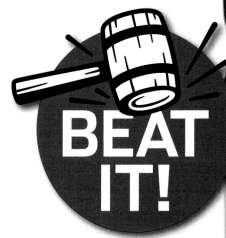

BEAT IT!

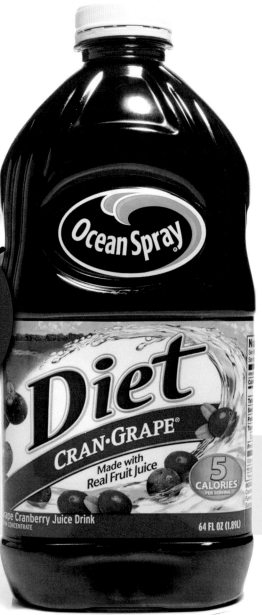

Sure, it's low in sugar, but it's also low in everything else, including actual juice. Instead, this is just flavored water with lots of artificial sweetener and chemical food dyes.

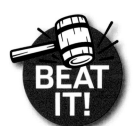

BEAT IT!

R.W. KNUDSEN
Very Veggie

60 calories
0 g fat
580 mg sodium
2 g fiber
8 g sugar
2 g protein

580 mg of sodium is a lot for 8 ounces of vegetable juice.

SUNNY DELIGHT

50 calories
0 fat
160 mg sodium
14 g sugar
0 protein

Not only are the first two ingredients water and corn syrup, this beverage also contains canola oil and corn starch (refreshing!), plus artificial sweeteners sucralose and neotame (a relative of aspartame), and artificial colors. Only 5 percent juice.

WELCH'S
Light Concord Grape Juice Beverage

45 calories
0 g fat
75 mg sodium
11 g sugar
0 protein

Uses the controversial sweetener sucralose, linked to bowel inflammation and DNA damage

V8
Splash Fruit Medley Flavored Beverage

80 calories
0 g fat
25 mg sodium
17 g sugar
0 g protein

Only 10 percent juice, contains sucralose and artificial color

NEWMAN'S OWN
Gorilla Grape Fruit Juice Cocktail

140 calories
0 g fat
140 mg sodium
0 g fiber
33 g sugar
0 g protein

This cocktail is mostly water and sugar.

SMOOTHIES:

V8
Splash Tropical Colada Smoothies Juice Drink

100 calories
0 g fat
50 mg sodium
1 g fiber
18 g sugar
3 g protein

DANACTIVE
Strawberry/Blueberry

70 calories
1 g fat
40 mg sodium
13 g sugar
3 g protein

Contains neither strawberries or blueberries. Says "contains 0 juice"

ODWALLA
Mango Tango

220 calories
1 g fat
15 mg sodium
2 g fiber
44 g sugar
0 g protein

Drinking 44 grams of sugar will not quench your thirst or satisfy your hunger.

ACTIVA
Prune Drink Smoothie

160 calories
3 g fat
75 mg sodium
0 fiber
25 g sugar
6 g protein

There's got to be a healthier way to get things moving than with 25 g of sugar.

NAKED PROTEIN ZONE
Banana Chocolate Smoothie

250 calories
1.5 g fat
170 mg sodium
1 g fiber
34 g sugar
16 g protein

High sugar, high calories

STONYFIELD FARM
Strawberry Smoothie

230 calories
3 g fat
150 mg sodium
<1 g fiber
38 g sugar
10 g protein

DUNKIN' DONUTS
Fruit Punch Coolata (large)

470 calories
0 fat
70 mg sodium
0 fiber
114 g sugar
0 protein

JAMBA JUICE
Aloha Pineapple Smoothie (power)

570 calories
2 g fat
70 mg sodium
5 g fiber
127 g sugar
7 g protein

BURGER KING
Tropical Mango

450 calories
1.5 g fat
95 mg sodium
85 g sugar
4 g protein

SMOOTHIE KING
Pomegranate Punch

396 calories
0 fat
1 mg sodium
1 g fiber
93 g sugar
0 protein

COLD STONE CREAMERY
Mango Pineapple

520 calories
4.5 g fat
240 mg sodium
2 g fiber
88 g sugar
2 g protein

MEXICAN FOOD

You've heard of Montezuma's Revenge? It originally referred to stomach problems people got when traveling in Mexico, supposedly the price we Old World–types paid for Cortez's defeat of the Aztecs. But Montezuma, wise-guy warrior, might have had bigger ideas: specifically, letting healthy bean, rice, and vegetable-based Mexican cuisine get all screwed up by American food marketers.

Nowadays, the food we think of as Mexican is a bastardized version of a once nutritious diet, loaded up with cheese and meat—and often, cheese-and-meat-like substances—and tossed into the deep fryer. The result: Every time you need to buy a bigger belt, an Aztec ancient laughs.

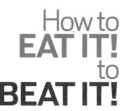

How to
EAT IT!
to
BEAT IT!

Much of the damage of a Mexican meal is done before the meal arrives—in the form of fried tortilla chips packed with salt. But that doesn't mean you can't order wisely and beat the Mexican stand-off.

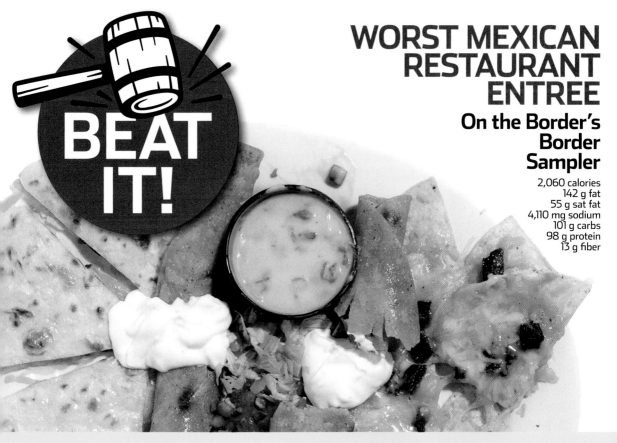

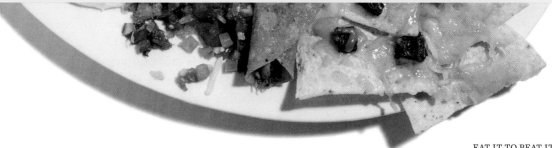

WORST MEXICAN RESTAURANT ENTREE

On the Border's Border Sampler

2,060 calories
142 g fat
55 g sat fat
4,110 mg sodium
101 g carbs
98 g protein
13 g fiber

On the Border of insanity, perhaps. This combo of chicken quesadillas, steak nachos, and chicken flautas equals a day's worth of calories and almost two day's worth of sodium.

THE MEXICAN RULES

GO FOR THE TACO. When eating Mexican food out at a restaurant, you're better off ordering a taco rather than a burrito. Most burritos hover around the 1,000-calorie mark, but you can find plenty of tacos out there for 300 calories.

BEAT THE WRAP. You may think that you're eating healthy because there's no bread on the table. But tortilla wraps, because they rely on fat to make them pliable, are actually higher in calories than bread.

GUAC SI, SOUR CREAM NO. Guacamole is loaded with calories, but it's also loaded with heart-healthy monounsaturated fats.

THAT'S NOT-CHO APPETIZER. Nachos are some of the highest calorie foods on every menu out there. Eat with caution and about 3 of your friends.

DON'T GET TOO "AUTHENTIC." Many Mexican restaurants have alternatives like grilled steaks or fish that don't include fatty tortillas. If you indulge in the chips beforehand, order a tortilla-free entree.

PLAY THE MAGICAL FRUIT. Eating more beans can help you lose belly fat and consume more vitamins, according to research in the *Journal of the American College of Nutrition*. Another study in *Advances in Nutrition* found that eating beans can help you feel more full after a meal, causing you to eat less, and lose weight. More of those, less of the nachos, okay?

HOW TO SPEAK MEXICAN

If it's on a tortilla that's fried, it's a tostada. If there's another tortilla on top, it's a quesa-dilla. If the tortil-la's folded, it's a taco. If it's rolled, it's a burrito. If it's rolled tightly, it's a taquito. If it's covered with sauce, it's an enchilada. If it's rolled tightly and covered with sauce, it's a flauta. So yes, it's all exactly the same, just like you thought.

The chicken filling is a mixture of white meat, dark meat, soy protein, water, and cornstarch; it contains something called "artificial sour cream flavor"; there are also trans fats ("partially hydrogenated cottonseed/soybean oil") and disodium EDTA (an additive made from cyanide and formaldehyde); MSG is there in 6 different forms, and it also contains propylene glycol (you know it as antifreeze; it's also the ingredient in electric cigarettes). The good news: You won't need to buy Junior that chemistry set for Christmas.

WORST MEXICAN SUPERMARKET ENTREE

Smart Ones Classic Favorites Chicken Enchiladas Suiza

290 calories
5 g fat
2 g sat fat
640 mg sodium
3 g fiber
4 g sugar
11 g protein

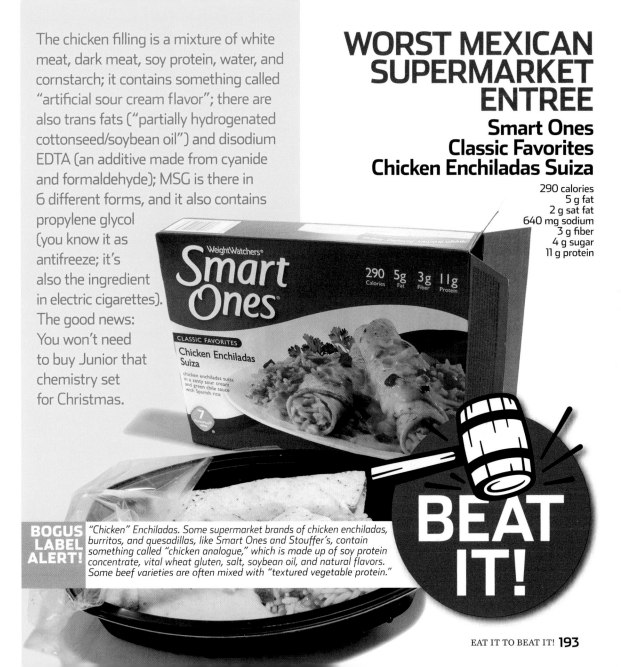

BOGUS LABEL ALERT! *"Chicken" Enchiladas. Some supermarket brands of chicken enchiladas, burritos, and quesadillas, like Smart Ones and Stouffer's, contain something called "chicken analogue," which is made up of soy protein concentrate, vital wheat gluten, salt, soybean oil, and natural flavors. Some beef varieties are often mixed with "textured vegetable protein."*

BEAT IT!

BEST MEXICAN RESTAURANT ENTREE

Baja Fresh Original Steak Taco

230 calories
8 g fat
2 g sat fat
260 mg sodium
2 g fiber

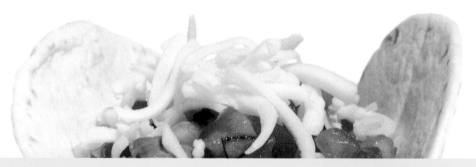

A chain restaurant dish with more protein than fat? Go ahead and eat two!

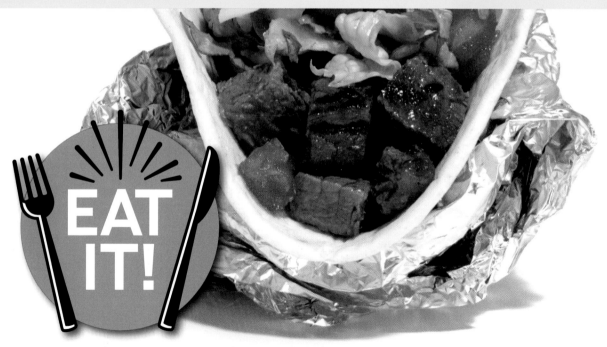

EAT IT!

CALIFORNIA PIZZA KITCHEN

White Corn Guacamole and Chips

- 360 calories
- 16 g fat
- 3 g sat fat
- 501 mg sodium
- 48 g carbs
- 3 g sugar
- 7 g fiber
- 6 g protein

TACO BELL

Fresco Burrito Supreme Steak

- 350 calories
- 9 g fat
- 3 g sat fat
- 1,020 mg sodium
- 6 g fiber
- 4 g sugar
- 18 g protein

Fresco Chicken Soft Taco

- 140 calories
- 3.5 g fat
- 1 g sat fat
- 470 mg sodium
- 2 g fiber
- 2 g sugar
- 10 g protein

CHIPOTLE

Steak Taco
(with salsa, lettuce, and cheese)

- 495 calories
- 21 g fat
- 8.5 g sat fat
- 1,000 mg sodium
- 5 g fiber
- 7 g sugar
- 42 g protein

Black Bean Burrito
(with brown rice, salsa, lettuce, and cheese)

- 695 calories
- 22.5 g fat
- 9 g sat fat
- 1,720 mg sodium
- 17 g fiber
- 4 g sugar
- 26 g protein

ON THE BORDER

Firecracker Stuffed Jalapeños
(with Original Queso)

- 1,910 calories
- 135 g fat
- 38 g sat fat
- 6,050 mg sodium
- 61 g protein
- 5 g fiber

Dos XX Fish Tacos
(with Creamy Red Chile Sauce)

- 1,950 calories
- 121 g fat
- 28 g sat fat
- 57 g protein
- 5 g fiber
- 3,540 mg sodium

BAJA FRESH

Steak Nacho Burrito

- 1,347 calories
- 50 g fat
- 21 g sat fat
- 81 g protein
- 22 g fiber
- 3,224 mg sodium

APPLEBEE'S

Sizzling Skillet Fajitas— Steak

- 1,330 calories
- 48 g fat
- 22 g sat fat
- 5,270 mg sodium
- 10 g fiber
- 77 g protein

TGI FRIDAY'S

Loaded Skillet Chip Nachos

- 1,520 calories
- 100 g fat
- 42 g sat fat
- 4,100 mg sodium
- 8 g fiber
- 53 g protein

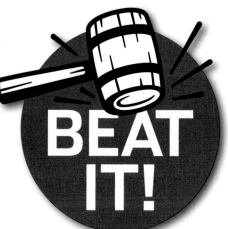

CHILI'S

Quesadilla Explosion Salad

- 1,430 calories
- 96 g fat
- 28 g sat fat
- 3,090 mg sodium
- 9 g fiber
- 14 g sugar
- 63 g protein

CHEESECAKE FACTORY

Factory Burrito Grande

- 1,839 calories
- 29 g sat fat
- 3,776 mg sodium

OUTBACK STEAKHOUSE

Alice Springs Chicken Quesadillas Regular

- 1,561 calories
- 97 g fat
- 42 g sat fat
- 3,095 mg sodium
- 4 g fiber
- 13 g sugar
- 88 g protein

BEST MEXICAN SUPERMARKET ENTREE

Helen's Kitchen Burrito Bowls Fiesta Black Bean Bowl

240 calories
8 g fat
3.5 g sat fat
380 mg sodium
8 g fiber
6 g sugar
12 g protein

Made with organic quinoa, spinach, and black beans. GMO free. No MSG, no artificial anything.

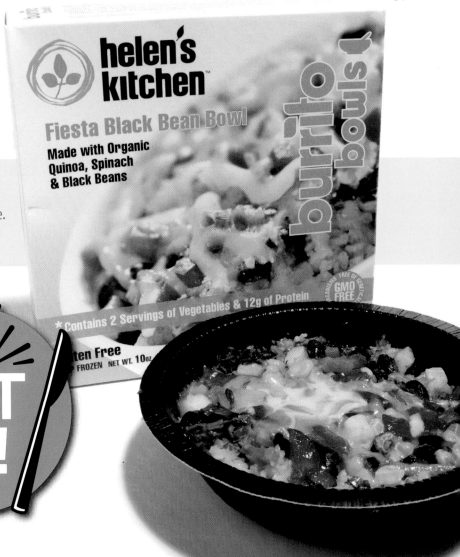

EAT IT!

AMY'S
Tamale Verde Black Bean
330 calories
10 g fat
780 mg sodium
12 g fiber
6 g sugar
7 g protein

RED'S
Burrito Steak
470 calories
11 g fat
510 mg sodium
6 g fiber
3 g sugar
29 g protein

AMY'S
Whole Meals Enchilada
(with Spanish Rice & Beans)
330 calories
8 g fat
1 g sat fat
740 mg sodium
9 g fiber
4 g sugar
9 g protein

CEDARLANE
Burrito Grande
(with Chili Verde Sauce)
230 calories
10 g fat
4 g sat fat
540 mg sodium
2 g fiber
3 g sugar
9 g protein

EVOL
Burrito Cilantro Lime Chicken
340 calories
11 g fat
210 mg sodium
4 g fiber
1 g sugar
15 g protein

KASHI
Entree Chicken Enchilada
280 calories
9 g fat
2.5 g sat fat
620 mg sodium
6 g fiber
5 g sugar
12 g protein

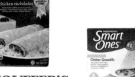

STOUFFER'S
Chicken Enchiladas
290 calories
9 g fat
5 g sat fat
740 mg sodium
3 g fiber
3 g sugar
13 g protein

Contains something called "chicken analogue," which is made up of soy protein concentrate, vital wheat gluten, salt, soybean oil, and natural flavors.

TGI FRIDAY'S
Quesadilla Rolls, Chicken
250 calories
12 g fat
4 g sat fat
410 mg sodium
2 g fiber
2 g sugar
10 g protein

Partially hydrogenated soybean oil and wood pulp (cellulose)

WEIGHT WATCHERS SMART ONES
Chicken Cheese Quesadilla
210 calories
6 g fat
2.5 g sat fat
470 mg sodium
7 g fiber
2 g sugar
11 g protein

MSG (hydrolyzed soy protein and autolyzed yeast extract), caramel color, cellulose

EL MONTEREY
Burritos, Beef & Bean
290 calories
14 g fat
5 g sat fat
340 mg sodium
3 g fiber
1 g sugar
9 g protein

Textured vegetable protein, caramel color, cellulose, and a little MSG (autolyzed yeast extract)

LAS CAMPANAS
Burritos, Beef & Bean
340 calories
15 g fat
530 mg sodium
3 g fiber
1 g sugar
9 g protein

Although there's beef in here, it is mixed with textured vegetable protein.

GOYA
Burrito, Beef 'n Bean (mild)
270 calories
6 g fat
2 g sat fat
530 mg sodium
0 g fiber
1 g sugar
14 g protein

Curious how something with beans in it can have zero fiber . . .

TINA'S
Burrito, Beef & Bean
280 calories
10 g fat
4 g sat fat
440 mg sodium
6 g fiber
2 g sugar
11 g protein

Textured vegetable protein mixed with the beef, wood pulp in the tortilla (cellulose)

NUT BUTTERS

What's sometimes smooth, sometimes gritty, really really rich, and usually attended by lots of lip-smacking? If you said Jay-Z and Beyoncé, good guess, but I was going for something a little more pedestrian.

There are few foods that can't be made better—healthier and yummier—by adding peanut butter or one of its close cousins, like cashew or almond butter. Loaded with fiber and heart-healthy monounsaturated fats, real, natural peanut butter is the world's most indulgent health food. And, if we were living in normal times, there would be no need for this chapter.

But these are not normal times, at least in the world of food. . . .

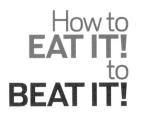

How to
EAT IT!
to
BEAT IT!

Picking the right nut butter comes down to only one rule: simplify. The fewer ingredients you have, the more nutrition you get.

GO ALTERNATIVE. Compared to peanut butter, almond butter has slightly fewer calories, twice the fiber, three more grams of healthy fat, and considerably less sodium. Almonds also contain more vitamin E, a powerful antioxidant.

What's "peanut butter spread"? Is it peanut butter that you, um, spread on stuff? Actually, according to the FDA, it's any vaguely peanut-butter-like product that's at least 10 percent additives, and hence can't legally be called "peanut butter." The healthiest peanut butters have one or two ingredients: peanuts, and maybe salt. But this Jif "spread" product has 15 ingredients, including corn syrup solids, molasses, and zinc oxide (yes, the stuff you rub on diaper rash).

WORST PEANUT BUTTER

Jif Reduced Fat Creamy Peanut Butter Spread

190 calories
12 g fat
2 g sat fat
6 g monounsaturated fat
220 mg sodium
2 g fiber
4 g sugar
7 g protein

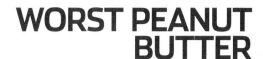

BEAT IT!

Sunflower seed butter has a similar nutritional profile, with a little less protein but higher levels of essential minerals.

GET FAT. "Reduced-fat" peanut butters are a lot like "reduced-fat" paychecks; thanks, but no thanks. Most peanut butters offer 2.5 grams of saturated fat and a whopping 13.5 grams of the good-for-you mono- and polyunsaturated fats. Reduced-fat peanut butter will reduce the saturated fat only by less than a gram, but will reduce the heart-healthy fats by about 30 percent.

DON'T TAKE JOY IN SOY. Soy nut butter is a good alternative for people with allergies to nuts (or if your child's school prohibits them). But all commercial brands we looked at had considerable amounts of sugar and other additives.

OR BE AMAZED BY HAZELNUT. Nutella may advertise itself as a healthy breakfast option, but it's really nothing more than chocolate cake icing. In fact, chocolate icing has 18 g of sugar per serving; Nutella has 21!

INVESTIGATE ORGANIC. Almost all the peanuts grown in the U.S. are treated with fungicides and pesticides, and residues are known to concentrate in oils. Especially if you eat a lot of peanut butter, buying organic is the easiest switch you can make to lessen exposure to toxic chemicals.

BOGUS LABEL ALERT! *The FDA allows products like Peter Pan, which contain less than 0.5 g of trans fats per serving, to say they're trans-fat free. But eat a little more than 2 tablespoons and you could be one-quarter of the way through your daily allowance for these cholesterol-raising bad-for-you fats.*

THE NUT BUTTER ADVANTAGE

Lose Weight

Although peanut butter is a high-calorie addition to celery sticks or what have you, all that protein, fiber, and healthy fat keeps you feeling full, allowing you to painlessly eat less. A 2013 study published in the *British Journal of Nutrition* found that peanut butter also increased levels of the hormone PYY, which is associated with appetite control.

Lower Blood Pressure

While some peanut butter is high in sodium, almost all is high in potassium—sodium's "good-guy" twin. Research has linked eating peanuts and peanut butter several times a week to having healthy blood pressure.

Lower Cholesterol

"Interventional studies consistently show that nut intake has a cholesterol-lowering effect," proclaimed a 2010 research review, "Health Benefits of Nut Consumption," in the journal *Nutrients*. That says it all, doesn't it?

Beat Diabetes

A recent study in the *British Journal of Nutrition* showed that eating peanuts or peanut butter during the day controlled blood sugar, even after a high-carb lunch. And an earlier study, from the *Journal of Nutrition* in 2009, showed that diabetics who eat peanut butter can significantly lower their risk for cardiovascular disease, a common diabetic complication.

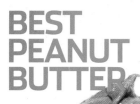

BEST PEANUT BUTTER

Smucker's Organic Natural Creamy

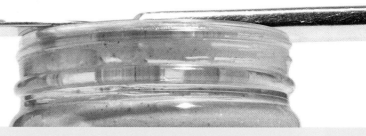

Ingredients: Peanuts, and less than 1 percent salt. Smucker's Natural line is a great choice.

210 calories
16 g fat
2.5 g sat fat
8 g monounsaturated fat
50 mg sodium
2 g fiber
1 g sugar
7 g protein

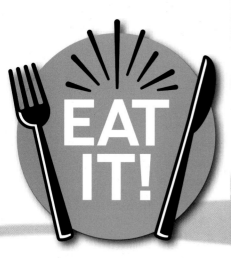

EAT IT!

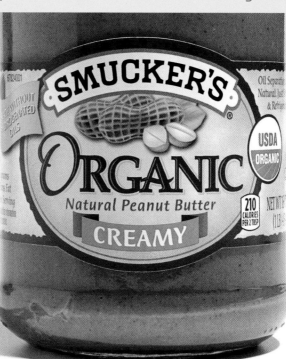

MARANATHA
Organic Peanut Butter Hint of Sea Salt Creamy

190 calories
16 g fat
2 g sat fat
80 mg sodium
3 g fiber
1 g sugar
8 g protein

100 percent organic dry roasted peanuts and sea salt. You can't get much better than that!

JUSTIN'S
Classic Almond Butter

200 calories
18 g fat
2 g saturated fat
0 mg sodium
4 g fiber
2 g sugar
7 g protein

Chocolate Hazelnut Butter

180 calories
15 g fat
3 g saturated fat
65 mg sodium
3 g fiber
7 g sugar,
4 g protein

The first two ingredients are hazelnuts and almonds.

JIF
Natural Peanut Butter Spread
(made with 90 percent peanuts)

190 calories
16 g fat
3 g saturated fat
80 mg sodium
2 g fiber
3 g sugar
7 g protein

Jif claims it's "natural," but by law it's not even all peanut butter: the qualifier "spread" means that the sugar, palm oil, and molasses added to this accounts for at least 10 percent of the ingredients.

Omega-3 Peanut Butter

190 calories
16 g fat
3 g saturated fat
150 mg sodium
2 g fiber
7 g protein
3 g sugar

Just as much added sugar, plus vegetable oils and fish oils

Chocolate Hazelnut Spread

230 calories
14 g fat
3.5 g saturated fat
40 mg sodium
21 g sugar
<1 g fiber
2 g protein

Jif recently got into the chocolate-hazelnut-spread business, and their version is even worse than Nutella. Two tablespoons of this spread has more sugar than a 5-ounce bag of Haribo Gold-Bears gummi bears.

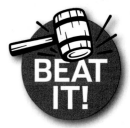

BEAT IT!

PETER PAN

210 calories
17 g fat
3 g saturated fat
140 mg sodium
3 g sugar
8 g protein
2 g fiber

Ingredients include partially hydrogenated oils (i.e. trans fats)

REESE'S
Creamy Peanut Butter

190 calories
16 g fat
2.5 g saturated fat
140 mg sodium
3 g fiber
8 g protein
3 g sugar

Contains sugar, hydrogenated oil, molasses, and cornstarch

SKIPPY
Creamy Peanut Butter

190 calories
16 g fat
3 g saturated fat
150 mg sodium
2 g fiber
3 g sugar
7 g protein

NUTRITION BARS

In this chapter, I want to tell you about one of my pet peeves: calorie bars.

You never heard of a "calorie bar" before? Well, you've heard of an "energy bar," right? Nutrition bars, protein bars, and meal replacement bars are often known by the catch-all "energy bars." And what is "energy"? It's calories. And that's what most nutrition bars are: tiny packages of calories.

Most of the bars out there are simply glorified candy all fancied up in nurse's uniforms and making racy nutrition claims—they're packed with fiber, they're full of protein, they're only 100 calories, blah blah blah. They sound healthy, but flip that label over and you'll see an ingredient list that looks like Charlie Sheen's blood test results.

Fortunately, several bars have come on the market in recent years with labels that don't read like a trick science question on

BOGUS LABEL ALERT!

"No trans fat." You'll be hard pressed to find a health bar out there that admits it has any trans fat in it. But when you look at the ingredient list for most bars, you will see partially hydrogenated oils. You'll also see something called "mechanically fractionated palm kernel oil." Some companies switched to palm oil when they were required to label trans fats. But researchers have found that palm oil, though not a trans fat, behaves in the body in exactly the same way, leading to dangerously high levels of LDL cholesterol and proteins in the blood. Offenders include: PowerBar, Special K, Kashi, Balance, Honey Stinger, and Zone, to name a few.

This bar might seem like a nice low-calorie protein bar, but when you take a look at what you're actually eating, it's clear that this is just an artificial candy bar. The "coating" is made with trans fats, soy, and sugar with a little cocoa processed with alkali, artificial flavor, polysorbate 60, and other ingredients.

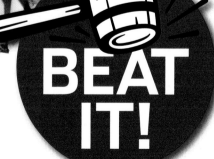

Kellogg's Special K Protein Meal Bar Double Chocolate

170 calories
4.5 g fat
200 mg sodium
5 g fiber
15 g sugar
10 g protein

And that's just the coating! Then there are the "Chocolatey Chips," which is market slang for "not real chocolate." Instead they are just more sugar, soy, trans fats, and artificial flavors mixed with a little alkalized cocoa.

BEAT IT!

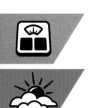

the SATs. Chose those, and you'll gain fiber, protein, and plenty of health-boosting vitamins and minerals. Here's how.

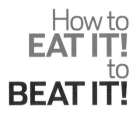

How to
EAT IT!
to
BEAT IT!

A quickly digested energy bar filled with sugar might make sense in some circumstances—for instance, you're cycling the Tour de France and your "special package" from the clinic in Florida hasn't arrived yet. But for most of us, calorie bars—I mean, "nutrition bars"—need to be taken with a grain of salt.

DOUBT THE NUMBERS. As a base, fewer than 250 calories is the first thing to look for. But a bar that looks good by the sugar/fiber/protein numbers can be hiding all sorts of artificial sweeteners, trans fats, and fake ingredients like "chocolaty chips." This is a case where it pays to skim the ingredients. The fewer, the better.

DON'T GO "-OL" IN. Some companies have replaced some of their sugar calories with sugar alcohols like maltitol and lactitol to decrease their overall calorie counts. But these syrups can cause bloating, gas, and have a laxative effect at high doses. Some Balance Bars, Pure Protein Bars, Atkins Breakfast Bars, and Slim-Fast 3-2-1 Plan Meal Bars contain them. As a result, foods that are packed with questionable chemicals appear to be lower in sugar.

KNOW YOUR CARB NEEDS. For a pre-workout bar you want about 40 grams of carbs. For a mid-day snack bar you need only about 15 g carbs.

DON'T SATURATE. There's no need for a bar to have more than 1 or 2 grams of saturated fat. And make sure the fat comes from healthy sources like nuts and seeds, not cloggy fats like hydrogenated oils, fractionated oils, palm oil, and the like.

HYDRATE. These bars are often condensed and a bit gooey and it's best to eat them with a generous amount of water so that they are more easily digested.

COOL IT WITH THE PROTEIN, ARNOLD. You don't need more than 20 grams of protein to recover from even the most strenuous workout. Mega-protein bars are just mega hype. In fact, a study in the *American Journal of Clinical Nutrition* found that 20 grams of intact protein is the ideal amount to facilitate muscle recovery after exercise. For everyday exercise, 6 grams of protein will do just fine.

THE NUTRITION BAR ADVANTAGE

Lose Weight

A recent study in the *Nutrition Journal* found that eating a grain-based nutrition bar (140 kcals, 25 g total carbohydrate, 3 g total fat, 0 g saturated fat, 2 g protein, 130 mg sodium, and 2 g fiber) before a meal, helped people feel fuller longer and lead to significant weight loss over time.

Improve Mood

Recent research on a group of Finnish military men found that eating a protein-rich energy bar helped them feel less hungry after a workout and improved their mood after training.

BEST NUTRITION BAR

KIND Fruit & Nut Bar
Nut Delight All Natural

200 calories
13 g fat
1.5 g sat fat
10 mg sodium
17 g carbs
3 g fiber
9 g sugar
9 g protein

This bar has little more than peanuts, almonds, brazil nuts, walnuts, honey, and a bit

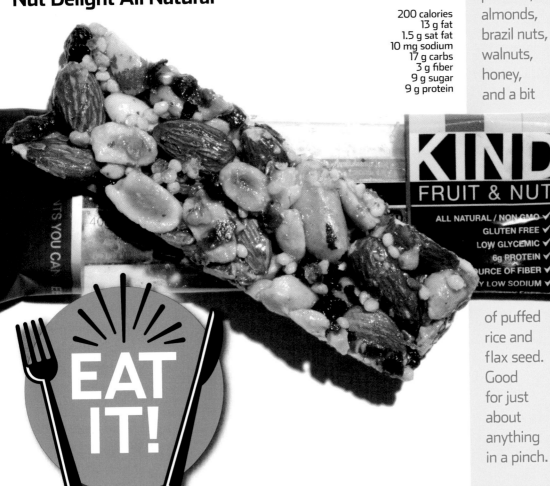

KIND®
FRUIT & NUT

ALL NATURAL / NON GMO ✓
GLUTEN FREE ✓
LOW GLYCEMIC ✓
6g PROTEIN ✓
URCE OF FIBER ✓
Y LOW SODIUM ✓

of puffed rice and flax seed. Good for just about anything in a pinch.

EAT IT!

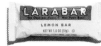

LARABAR

Food Bar, Lemon Bar

220 calories
11 g fat
1.5 g sat fat
5 mg sodium
28 g carbs
3 g fiber
22 g sugar
6 g protein

Simply contains dates, cashews, almonds, lemon juice concentrate, natural lemon flavor

Apple Pie

190 calories
10 g fat
1 g sat fat
5 mg sodium
24 g carbs
5 g fiber
18 g sugar
4 g protein

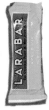

CLIFF BAR

Crunchy Peanut Butter

250 calories
6 g fat
1 g sat fat
240 mg sodium
41 g carbs
4 g fiber
21 g sugar
11 g protein

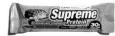

SUPREME PROTEIN

Carb Conscious 15g Protein Bar Caramel Nut Chocolate

200 calories
8 g fat
5 g sat fat
150 mg sodium
18 g carbs
<1 g fiber
5 g sugar
15 g protein

5 times as much saturated fat as fiber

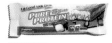

PURE PROTEIN

Bar S'mores

180 calories
5 g fat
3.5 g sat fat
130 mg sodium
20 g carbs
0 g fiber
2 g sugar
19 g protein

*Maltitol, fractionated palm kernel oil . . . and sucralose is listed not once but twice.
A study in* Diabetes Care *found that this artificial sweetener can affect blood insulin levels much the same way as sugar can.*

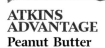

ATKINS ADVANTAGE

Peanut Butter Granola Bar

210 calories
11 g fat
3 g sat fat
240 mg sodium
18 g carbs
5 g fiber
1 g sugar
15 g protein

Maltitol, palm kernel and palm oil, partially defatted peanut flour . . . Have some peanuts instead.

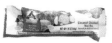

Caramel Chocolate Nut Roll

180 calories
12 g fat
5 g sat fat
200 mg sodium
20 g carbs
8 g fiber
2 g sugar
8 g protein

Maltitol, palm kernel oil, plus artificial flavors and sucralose

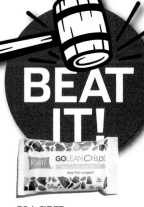

KASHI

GOLEAN Crisp! Bar Chocolate Almond

170 calories
5 g fat
2.5 g sat fat
210 mg sodium
27 g carbs
5 g fiber
13 g sugar
8 g protein

Mechanically fractionated palm kernel oil

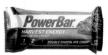

POWERBAR

ProteinPlus Bar Chocolate Crisp

210 calories
5 g fat
3 g sat fat
120 mg sodium
27 g carbs
4 g fiber
12 g sugar
20 g protein

"Chocolate Flavored Coating"—i.e., Something other than chocolate

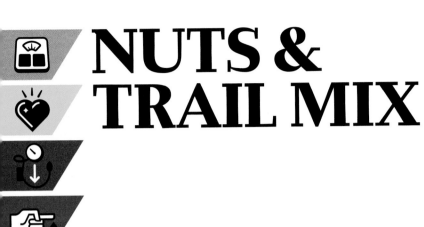

NUTS & TRAIL MIX

If a reliable doctor gave you a weight-loss pill, would you take it?

How about a second pill to lower your blood pressure? Another to manage cholesterol? Another to fight diabetes? One more to make sure you got all your vitamins? You'd start to feel like a walking Walgreens.

But what if, instead of turning your bathroom into a set piece for *Celebrity Rehab,* you could get all those benefits from popping just one pill—one chewable, delicious, and all-natural pill? Well, that's what nuts are: nature's original multivitamin.

In fact, nuts are so propitiously packed with power that modern food packagers just couldn't resist finding a way to screw them up. You could always go hunting for wild hickory nuts, but if foraging in the woodlands isn't your thing, then try this approach to healthy nut-trition.

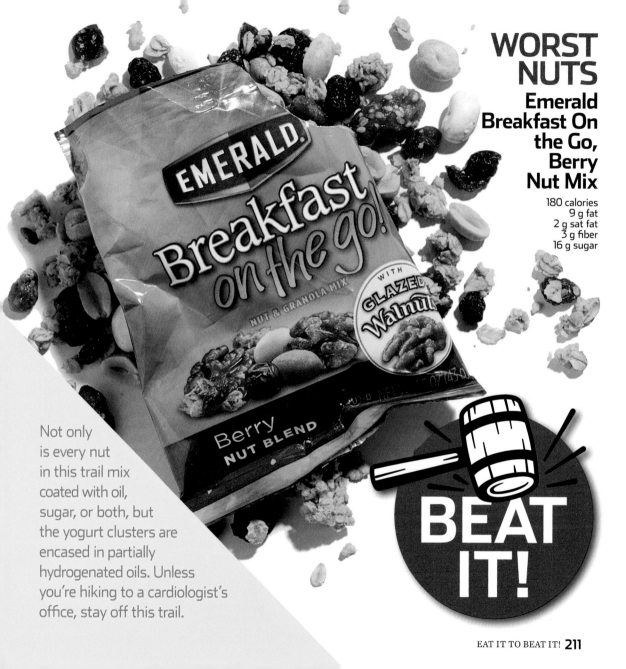

WORST NUTS

Emerald Breakfast On the Go, Berry Nut Mix

180 calories
9 g fat
2 g sat fat
3 g fiber
16 g sugar

Not only is every nut in this trail mix coated with oil, sugar, or both, but the yogurt clusters are encased in partially hydrogenated oils. Unless you're hiking to a cardiologist's office, stay off this trail.

BEAT IT!

How to
EAT IT!
to
BEAT IT!

Take fresh, healthy nuts, roast them in oil, coat them with salt, throw them into a bag with lots of sugar, and what do you have? The Trail Mix of Tears. Here's how to stay on the right path.

THE MIX RULES

GO RAW. Roasted nuts are usually roasted in vegetable oils, which means they've added unhealthy fats on top of the healthy ones. Raw or dry-roasted nuts are a healthy alternative.

SPIKE THE SUGAR. Too many trail mixes are loaded with candies or "fruit" that came right out of Willie Wonka's nightmare. Look for less than 3 grams sugar per serving.

THE NUTTY PROFESSOR

How to be an instant expert in the shell game.

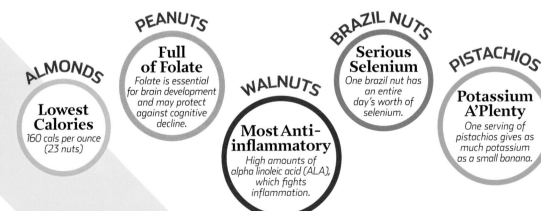

ALMONDS
Lowest Calories
160 cals per ounce (23 nuts)

PEANUTS
Full of Folate
Folate is essential for brain development and may protect against cognitive decline.

WALNUTS
Most Anti-inflammatory
High amounts of alpha linoleic acid (ALA), which fights inflammation.

BRAZIL NUTS
Serious Selenium
One brazil nut has an entire day's worth of selenium.

PISTACHIOS
Potassium A'Plenty
One serving of pistachios gives as much potassium as a small banana.

THE NUT MIX ADVANTAGE

Lose Weight

A large review of peanuts and tree nuts' effect on weight published in 2008 in the *Journal of Nutrition* concluded that nuts can be included in a diet without any negative effect on weight and may even be helpful. Another study published in 2011 in the *Journal of the American College of Nutrition* found that people who eat tree nuts have decreased BMIs and waist circumference.

Beat Diabetes

The same study in the *Journal of the American College of Nutrition* linked consumption of tree nuts to lower diabetes risk.

Lower Cholesterol

All nuts contain fiber, which helps lower your cholesterol. A review from Loma Linda University published in 2010 pooled data from 25 studies in seven countries and found that daily nut intake lowered cholesterol on average by 5.1 percent.

Lower Blood Pressure

A study published in 2013 in the journal *Nutrients* found that a diet that included nuts was inversely associated with high blood pressure.

BEST NUTS
Blue Diamond Sea Salt Oven Roasted Almonds

The primary fat in almonds is mono-unsaturated fat, which has been shown to help lower cholesterol and control weight gain. These almonds have a touch of salt and a dash of sweet, to help keep you satiated and coming back for more.

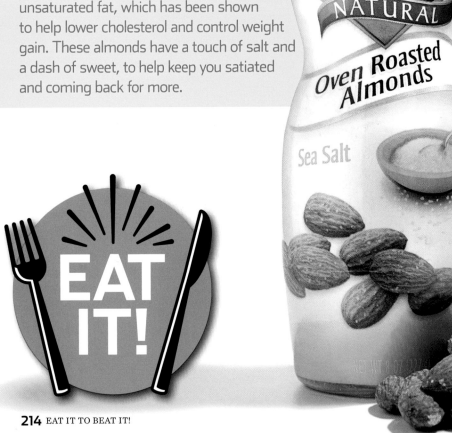

170 calories
15 g fat
1 g sat fat
135 mg sodium
3 g fiber
1 g sugar
6 g protein
24 nuts

EAT IT!

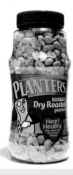

PLANTERS
Regular Unsalted Peanuts

170 calories
14 g fat
2 g sat fat
5 mg sodium
2 g fiber
1 g sugar
8 g protein

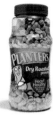

PLANTERS
Regular Dry-Roasted Peanuts

170 calories
14 g fat
2 g sat fat
160 mg sodium
2 g sugar
2 g fiber
7 g protein

Sugar and corn syrup

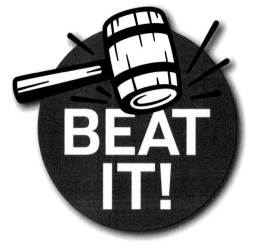

BEAT IT!

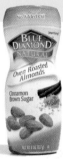

BLUE DIAMOND
Cinnamon Brown Sugar Almonds

160 calories
14 g fat
1 g sat fat
30 mg sodium
3 g fiber
3 g sugar
6 g protein

Even though they're sweetened, they kept the sugar content low. Nice job, guys!

NUT-rition Antioxidant Mix

160 calories
11 g fat
3 g sat fat
0 mg sodium
2 g fiber
11 g sugar
4 g protein

Despite the health claims of Planters special nutrition mixes, they're mostly loaded with sugar and vegetable oils.

EMERALD
Sweet & Salty Mixed Nut Blend Original

150 calories
12 g fat
1.5 g sat fat
115 mg sodium
2 g fiber
5 g sugar
5 g protein

Almost every nut is mixed with sugar, corn syrup, and oil.

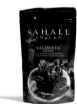

SAHALE
Valdosta Pecans

130 calories
11 g fat
1 g sat fat
50 mg sodium
2 g fiber
7 g sugar
1 g protein
1/4 cup

Sugar is in the ingredient list 4 different ways: sugar, evaporated cane juice, organic tapioca syrup, and brown sugar.

PASTA & PASTA DISHES

For most of American history, pasta was to dinner what Ringo Starr was to the Beatles: a goofy, bland, but reliable backup player supporting an exciting trio of meat, vegetables, and sauce. And like Ringo, when you have it alone, it's just kinda . . . blah.

But lately, pasta has gotten complicated. Caught between the whole-grain craze and the gluten-free craze, food marketers have been working hard to improve their basic refined-wheat-and-water recipes. But in reality, it matters more what you put on your pasta than what the noodles themselves are made of. Want proof? The average American man eats 19.4 pounds of pasta a year. The average Italian man eats 57.3 pounds of pasta a year. The average American man weighs 191 pounds. The average Italian man: 160.

BOGUS LABEL ALERT!

"Protected carbs." Dreamfields pasta claims to have patented a method of suspending the starch in their pastas so that it doesn't affect blood sugar levels. A box of their spaghetti has 41 grams of carbohydrates, but they claim that 31 of those grams are "protected carbs" that won't break down in the body, leaving only 5 digestible grams of carbs. However, the one study that did try to replicate their claims found that blood glucose levels spiked in exactly the same way that they do with regular pasta.

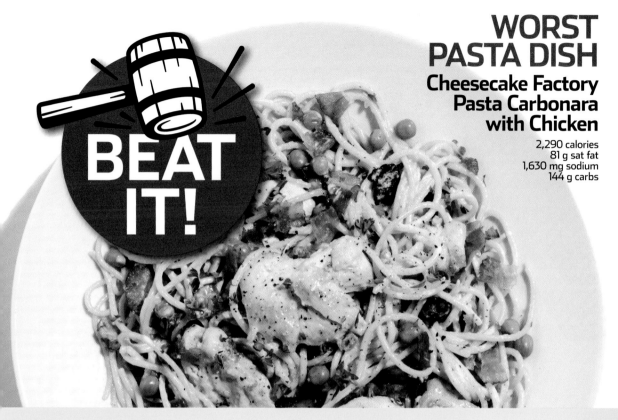

WORST PASTA DISH

Cheesecake Factory Pasta Carbonara with Chicken

2,290 calories
81 g sat fat
1,630 mg sodium
144 g carbs

BEAT IT!

It's not the pasta itself that really matters, but what the pasta wears when it goes out to dinner. In this case, Cheesecake Factory has dressed their innocent little spaghetti noodles in a fat suit: Not only does this dish have more calories than most of us should eat in a day, it has the saturated fat equivalent of 1 1/3 sticks of butter—or half a dozen bratwursts.

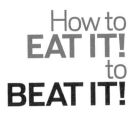

How to
EAT IT!
to
BEAT IT!

THE PASTA RULES

KEEP IT SIMPLE. All you need to make good pasta is wheat, water, and salt. When you see things like gum gluten, disodium phosphate (to shorten cooking time), glyceryl monostearate, and various dyes and colorings, use your noodle—and choose something else.

GO WHOLE GRAIN. Or try a different kind of blend, like Barilla Plus, which is made with semolina flour but is blended with legumes, lentils, chickpeas, flaxseeds, barley, and other ingredients that are far better for you than just plain pasta. When picking a whole-grain pasta, you should see the word "whole" somewhere near the wheat listed in the ingredients.

DON'T GUM IT UP. Once you overcook pasta, it gets all gummy and starchy, and even whole-wheat pastas will break down quicker in your stomach. That's one reason they tell you to cook pasta al dente (to the tooth)—it's not only tastier, but healthier for you!

THE PASTA ADVANTAGE

Boost Immunity
Researchers from the University of Scranton in Pennsylvania found that foods like pasta contain polpyhenols, a healthy antioxidant, and that whole-grain products have comparable antioxidants per gram to fruits and vegetables.

Beat Diabetes

A 2008 study by the Department of Clinical and Experimental Medicine in Naples, Italy, found that foods like whole-wheat pasta, with a low glycemic index—the measurement of how quickly blood sugar rises after food intake—and high-fiber content could control blood glucose and protect against diabetes.

Lose Weight

A study conducted in Northern Sweden found that pasta eaters had a more favorable fat distribution around the waistline. And a Harvard Medical School and Brigham and Women's Hospital study found that women who ate high-fiber, whole-grain foods were 49 percent less likely to gain weight.

Improve Mood

Researchers at MIT found that cutting out carbohydrates like pasta reduces levels of the happiness hormone serotonin, a chemical that suppresses appetite.

Lower Blood Pressure

Some whole-wheat pasta can have around 7 grams of fiber and 8 ounces of protein per 2-ounce serving. A study at the University of Western Australia found that high-protein, high-fiber diets can lower blood pressure.

Lower Cholesterol

Researchers in France confirmed that a healthy diet full of whole-grain, high-fiber foods, like pasta, especially when consumed early in life, can lower LDL cholesterol by 5 to 10 percent.

BIZARRE WEIGHT-LOSS TRICK

Want to gain less weight from a serving of pasta? Put it in the fridge. Chilling pasta changes the nature of the starch in the noodles, making it into something called "resistant starch," meaning your body has to work harder to digest it. Colder noodles = hotter you.

BEST PASTA DISH

Carrabba's Italian Grill Spaghetti Pomodoro with Whole Grain Spaghetti

431 calories
4 g fat
1 g sat fat
1,416 mg sodium
18 g fiber
6 g sugar
18 g protein

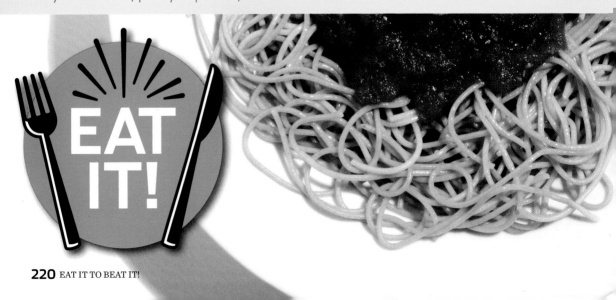

Although the sodium is a bit high for my liking, this dish has about two-thirds of your daily fiber needs, plenty of protein, and lots of vitamins and minerals from the sauce.

EAT IT!

OLIVE GARDEN
Whole Wheat Linguini Pomodoro
(you have to ask for the whole wheat)

- 490 calories
- 11 g fat
- 2 g sat fat
- 965 mg sodium
- 11 g fiber
- 18 g protein

ROMANO'S MACARONI GRILL
Whole Wheat Fettuccine Pomodoro
(create Your Own Pasta)

- 680 calories
- 17 g fat
- 2.5 g sat fat
- 1,280 mg sodium
- 19 g fiber
- 30 g protein

CARRABBA'S ITALIAN GRILL
Linguini Pescatore with Whole Grain Spaghetti

- 702 calories
- 7 g fat
- 1 g sat fat
- 2,048 mg sodium
- 18 g fiber
- 9 g sugar
- 63 g protein

Whole-grain pasta having a party with omega-3-rich seafood. Not a good choice if you're watching your sodium, but this dish packs a one-two punch of protein and fiber that's hard to beat.

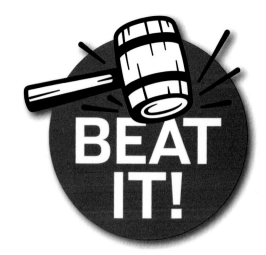

OLIVE GARDEN
Five Cheese Ziti al Forno

- 1,170 calories
- 55 g fat
- 30 g sat fat
- 2,090 mg sodium
- 10 g fiber
- 47 g protein

APPLEBEE'S
Three Cheese Chicken Penne

- 1,000 calories
- 46 g fat
- 24 g sat dfat
- 1 g trans fat
- 2,490 mg sodium
- 6 g fiber
- 57 g protein

BERTUCCI'S
Spaghetti with Meatballs Bolognese

- 1,880 calories
- 84 g fat
- 35 g sat fat
- 3,740 mg sodium
- 11 g fiber
- 86 g protein

CHILI'S
Cajun Pasta with Grilled Chicken

- 1,300 calories
- 62 g fat
- 4,630 mg sodium!!
- 8 g fiber
- 73 g protein

DOMINO'S
Pasta Primavera in a Bread Bowl

- 1,340 cal
- 48 g fat
- 22 g sat fat
- 1,760 mg sodium
- 8 g fiber
- 10 g sugar

BEST SUPERMARKET PASTA
DeLallo Capellini No. 1

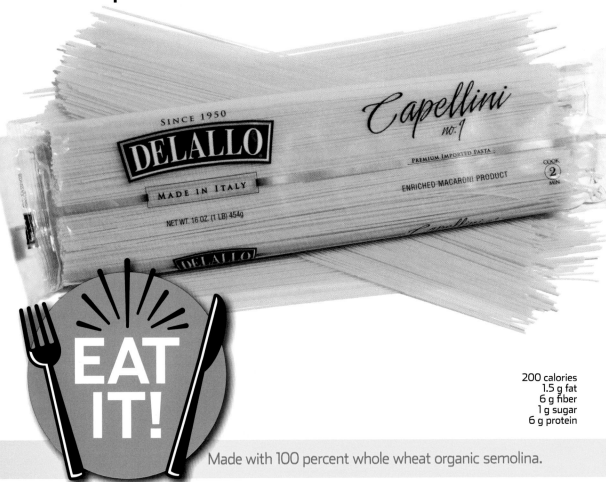

SINCE 1950

DELALLO.

MADE IN ITALY

NET WT. 16 OZ. (1 LB) 454g

Capellini no. 1

PREMIUM IMPORTED PASTA

ENRICHED MACARONI PRODUCT

COOK 2 MIN

200 calories
1.5 g fat
6 g fiber
1 g sugar
6 g protein

EAT IT!

Made with 100 percent whole wheat organic semolina.

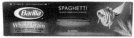

BARILLA
Whole Grain
- 200 calories
- 1.5 g fat
- 6 g fiber
- 7 g protein

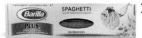

Plus
- 210 calories
- 2 g fat
- 4 g fiber
- 10 g protein

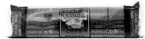

RACCONTA
8 Whole Wheat Capellini/ Angel Hair
- 210 calories
- 1 g fat
- 6 g fiber
- 7 g protein

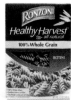

RONZONI
Healthy Harvest 100% Whole Wheat
- 180 calories
- 1.5 g fat
- 5 g fiber
- 9 g protein

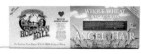

HODGSON MILL
Angel Hair, Whole Wheat, Whole Grain
- 210 calories
- 1 g fat
- 6 g fiber
- 9 g protein

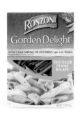

RONZONI
Garden Delight
- 200 calories
- 1 g fat
- 2 g fiber
- 8 g protein

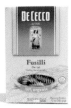

DE CECCO
100% Organic Fusilli
- 200 calories
- 1 g fat
- 2 g fiber
- 7 g protein

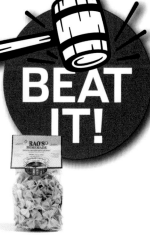

RAO'S
Te-Colori Farfalle
- 197 calories
- 1 g fat
- 2 g fiber
- 6 g protein

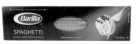

BARILLA
Spaghetti
- 200 calories
- 1 g fat
- 2 g fiber
- 7 g protein

BOGUS LABEL ALERT!

"Spinach" pasta does not count as a vegetable, no matter what the label claims. Ronzoni says their Garden Delight pasta gives you "half a serving of vegetables in each 2 ounce portion," and they show brightly colored spinach, tomatoes, and carrots on their label. But a 200-calorie serving of their Rotini gives you just 4 percent of your vitamin A, zero vitamin C, and only 2 percent of your calcium intake for the day. An actual ½ serving of real spinach, on the other hand (about ½ cup cooked), gives you nearly 50 times as much vitamin A and 12 times as much calcium—for only 20 calories.

PIZZA

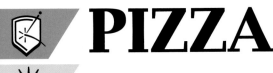

BOGUS LABEL ALERT!

Apparently zeroing in on just how lonely overeating can be, many restaurants have their own "individual" pizzas that test the limits of what one person's body can handle. Round Table has several "individual" size flatbreads, but a close look at their nutritional information tells us there are 4 servings per "individual" order! The King Arthur Supreme personal pizza is 180 calories per slice. But the whole personal pizza is 720 calories!

Back in 2009, Pizza Hut, the country's largest pizza chain, announced it was going "natural."

Fortunately, that didn't mean delivery guys would start showing up in the buff. No, the company instead garnered a ton of media attention for doing what no other fast food pizza chain was willing to do: cut out high fructose corn syrup, artificial preservatives, nitrates, and fillers. They even announced the launch of a new pizza called "The Natural," complete with a whole-grain crust.

Health advocates applauded the new pizza, nutrition-conscious pizza lovers rejoiced, and we all lived happily ever after. For about a year. By 2010, Pizza Hut had quietly stopped selling it.

This story is sad, but telling. Why would a company that sells food need to announce it's going "natural"? Isn't food supposed to be "natural" already? And pizza—at least in the form imagined by generations of Italian grandmothers—should already be a healthy, nutrition-packed meal. Well, at least it used to be. Until America's food companies got ahold of it.

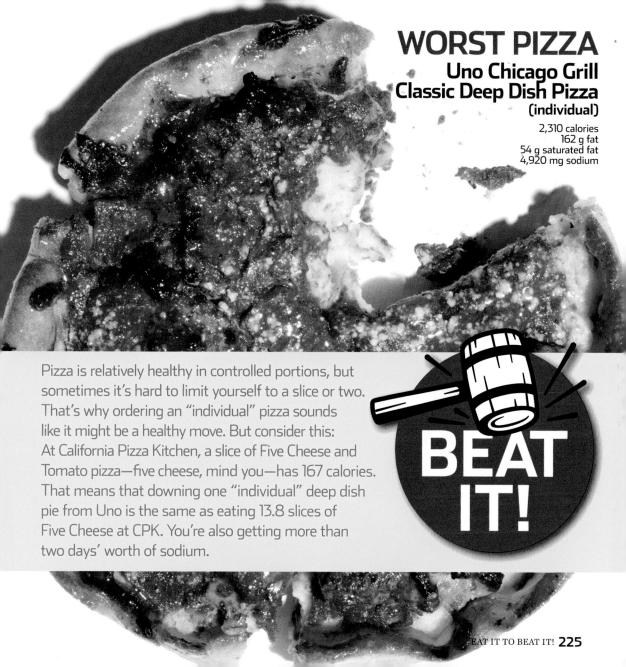

WORST PIZZA
Uno Chicago Grill
Classic Deep Dish Pizza
(individual)

2,310 calories
162 g fat
54 g saturated fat
4,920 mg sodium

Pizza is relatively healthy in controlled portions, but sometimes it's hard to limit yourself to a slice or two. That's why ordering an "individual" pizza sounds like it might be a healthy move. But consider this: At California Pizza Kitchen, a slice of Five Cheese and Tomato pizza—five cheese, mind you—has 167 calories. That means that downing one "individual" deep dish pie from Uno is the same as eating 13.8 slices of Five Cheese at CPK. You're also getting more than two days' worth of sodium.

BEAT IT!

How to
EAT IT!
to
BEAT IT!

One day, approximately 7,000 years ago, someone living along the Mediterranean looked at a boring piece of flat bread and thought, "I bet this would taste great with some toppings." (Which led, about 6,999 years ago, to the first war over whether or not to include anchovies.)

And in its first iterations, pizza was a relatively healthy meal: whole-grain bread, fresh cheese, tomato sauce, and plenty of herbs and vegetables gave you a complete meal with relatively few calories—a primitive food pyramid on a plate. Then American food manufacturers stepped in to "improve" this traditional Italian pie, and all hell broke loose. By dousing the crust in salt and oil, we managed to make a healthy meal into a carb crash that has us straining at our seat belts.

As a result, any plain pizza's health profile is a matter of balance between the toppings—cancer-fighting tomato sauce, bone-building cheese, and whatever healthy toppings you want to add—and the crust, where a remarkable number of sins can be committed. (You already know that by adding pepperoni or sausage to the pie, you're pretty much giving up any claim to "eating healthy." Each individual round of pepperoni has 10 calories, so every time you eat two slices, you're adding about 150 calories to your intake. Order pizza just once a week, and that pepperoni will add two pounds to your frame in a year. Now do that for the next ten years and see what happens.)

THE PIZZA RULES

DON'T BE PLAIN. One important aspect of controlling your weight is to avoid foods that are high on the Glycemic Index (GI), a measure of how quickly blood glucose levels rise in response

WORST FROZEN PIZZA
Totino's Mexican Style Party Big Party Pizza

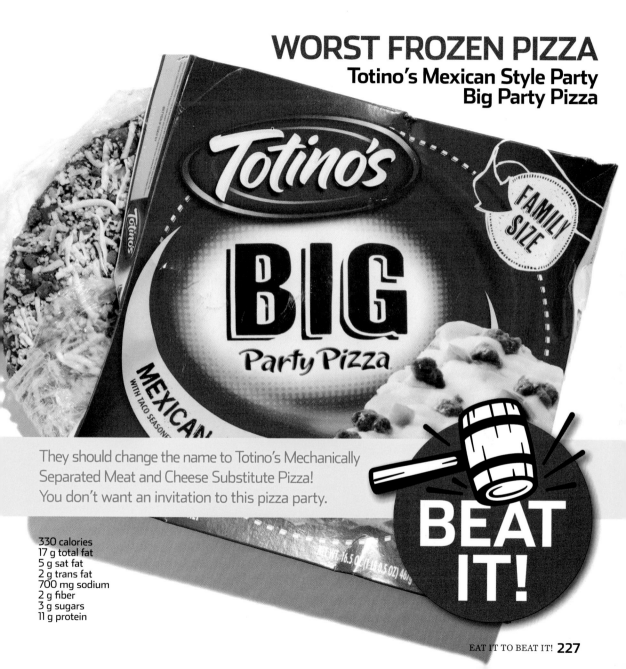

They should change the name to Totino's Mechanically Separated Meat and Cheese Substitute Pizza! You don't want an invitation to this pizza party.

330 calories
17 g total fat
5 g sat fat
2 g trans fat
700 mg sodium
2 g fiber
3 g sugars
11 g protein

BEAT IT!

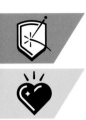

to a certain food with a measure of 1 to 100. The lower the score, the better. A simple cheese and tomato sauce pizza scores an 80, and a fully loaded Supreme pizza scores a 36 because of the added fat and protein. GI scores are only a suggestion of what to eat and what to avoid, but this suggests that plain cheese pizza isn't really doing you any good—the more vegetable toppings, the fuller and more satisfied you'll feel and the less pizza you will eat. Even lean meats, like chicken or ham, can add to your pizza's health benefits.

SEE RED. The biggest health benefits from pizza come from lycopene-rich tomato sauce. (Lycopene is a nutrient found in red foods like tomatoes and watermelon that's shown to reduce your risk of certain cancers.) White pizzas sacrifice the biggest health benefit of a traditional pie.

MAKE YOURSELF WHOLE. Some pizza joints offer whole-grain versions of their pizzas, which is just about the most delicious way to sneak extra fiber and nutrients into your diet.

PREPARE FOR A SALT. The biggest problem with American pizza is sodium content. Even the healthiest options can have up to 400 mg of sodium per slice, which means that a two-slice serving will give you nearly half a day's worth of salt. If you're salt sensitive, limit yourself to one slice.

GO FLAT. Most of the evils of pizza lie in the crust, so the less crust you indulge in, the better. That means thin-crust pizzas are almost always the better option. That said, even thin crusts tend to be loaded with sodium.

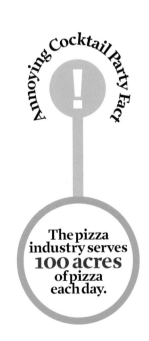

Annoying Cocktail Party Fact

The pizza industry serves **100 acres** of pizza each day.

Look at those nice Sbarro folks, offering up a healthy slice for mall shoppers everywhere! But don't be fooled; you can put a stick of asparagus on a doughnut, but it's still a doughnut. And eating two slices of Sbarro's "healthy" offering is the same as eating 5 Chocolate Iced Glazed doughnuts from Krispy Kreme, and more than a day's worth of sodium.

WORST "HEALTHY" PIZZA

Sbarro's Broccoli Spinach & Tomato Pan Pizza

640 calories
30 g fat
8 g sat fat
1,300 mg sodium
(per slice)

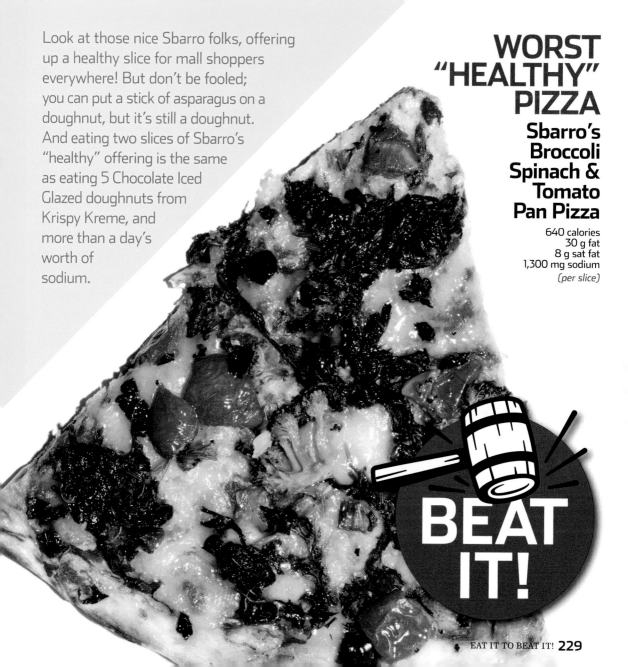

BEAT IT!

THE PIZZA ADVANTAGE

 Boost Immunity

One of the biggest sources of tomato-based ingredients in the American diet is pizza. Lycopene, the health-giving antioxidant in tomatoes, has been linked to a reduced risk of heart disease and cancer in epidemiological studies. It's thought that this is in part due to improving immune function, but more studies are needed. However, you can load your pizza with any and all kinds of vegetable toppings to get those immunity benefits. Recent studies have found that getting at least 5 servings of vegetables a day significantly reduces the risk of infection or illness in older adults.

Lower Cholesterol

Eating a lot of tomato-based products, including pizza, may help your cholesterol. A 2012 study from the *Journal of Nutrition* found that women who ate more than 10 servings of tomato-based foods per week (sauces, juices, whole tomatoes, and pizza) had modest improvements in total cholesterol and better ratios of HDL or "good" cholesterol and LDL or "bad" cholesterol. A 2012 study in the journal *Neurology* echoed these results when researchers found that eating lycopene-rich, tomato-based foods reduces your risk for stroke, in part by reducing cholesterol and preventing blood clots.

THE BEST HEALTHY PIZZA

Pizza Hut Hand-Tossed Veggie Lovers

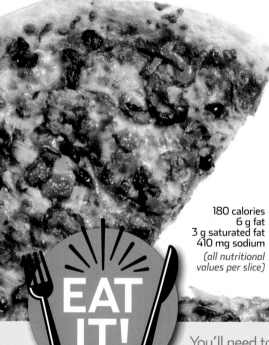

180 calories
6 g fat
3 g saturated fat
410 mg sodium

(all nutritional values per slice)

DOMINO'S
Brooklyn Style Crust Chorizo, Mushroom, Onion and Roasted Red Pepper Pizza

260 calories
11 g fat
645 mg sodium

PAPA JOHN'S
Garden Fresh Thin Crust Pizza

220 calories
11 g fat
360 mg sodium

CALIFORNIA PIZZA KITCHEN
Five Cheese and Tomato (thin crust)

139 calories
5.8 g fat
338 mg sodium

CICI'S PIZZA
Bacon Cheddar (to-go slice)

144 calories
7.6 g fat
408 mg sodium

BEAT IT!

PIZZA HUT
Veggie Lover's Personal PANormous Pizza (small)

1,010 calories
38 g fat
2,250 mg sodium

DOMINOS
Brooklyn Style Crust Sausage Pizza

660 calories
36 g fat
1,660 mg sodium

PAPA JOHN'S
Hawaiian BBQ Chicken Pizza

290 calories
13 g fat
680 mg sodium

CICI'S PIZZA
BBQ (to-go slice)

248 calories
6.6 g fat
450 mg sodium

CALIFORNIA PIZZA KITCHEN
Original Crust Margherita Pizza

610 calories
12 g fat
1,118 mg sodium
4 g fiber
18 g sugar
18 g protein

EAT IT!

You'll need to exercise Pizza Hut's "made to order" option, but we chose the hand-tossed pie over Pizza Hut's thin-crust option. With the same number of calories per slice, the hand-tossed delivers less sodium, less sugar and more protein than its thinner cousin.

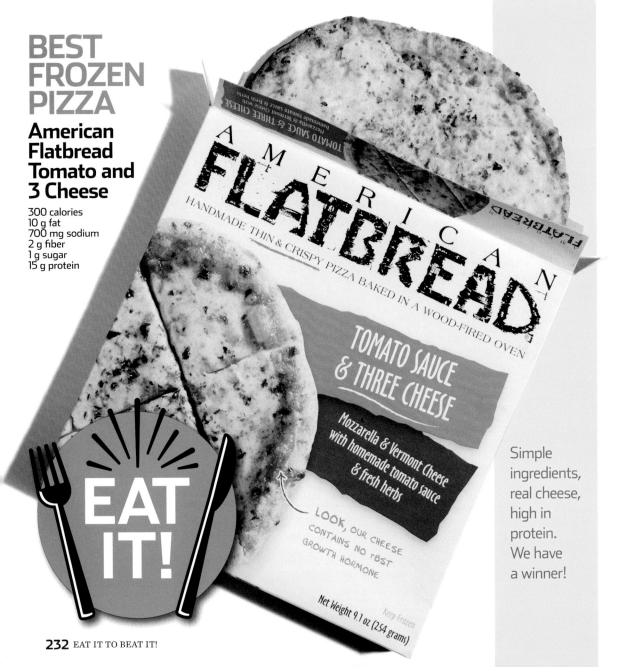

BEST FROZEN PIZZA

American Flatbread Tomato and 3 Cheese

300 calories
10 g fat
700 mg sodium
2 g fiber
1 g sugar
15 g protein

AMERICAN FLATBREAD

HANDMADE THIN & CRISPY PIZZA BAKED IN A WOOD-FIRED OVEN

TOMATO SAUCE & THREE CHEESE

Mozzarella & Vermont Cheese with homemade tomato sauce & fresh herbs

LOOK, OUR CHEESE CONTAINS NO rBST GROWTH HORMONE

EAT IT!

Simple ingredients, real cheese, high in protein. We have a winner!

Net Weight 9.1 oz (254 grams) Keep Frozen

WEGMANS
Thin Crust Cheese Pizza

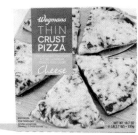

- 300 calories
- 11 g fat
- 700 mg sodium
- 2 g fiber
- 4 g sugar
- 13 g protein

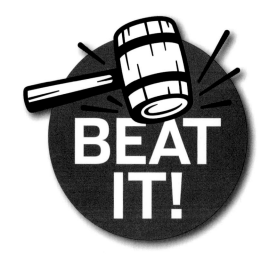

KASHI
Margherita, Thin Crust Pizza

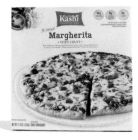

- 260 calories
- 9 g fat
- 630 mg sodium
- 4 g fiber
- 4 g sugar
- 14 g protein

DIGIORNO
Rising Crust Pepperoni Pizza

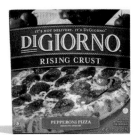

- 330 calories
- 13 g fat
- 940 mg sodium
- 2 g fiber
- 6 g sugar
- 14 g protein

Contains mechanically separated chicken (pink slime!) and nitrites

NEWMAN'S OWN
Thin & Crispy, Four Cheese Pizza

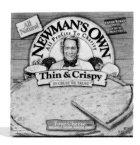

- 300 calories
- 13 g fat
- 610 mg sodium
- 2 g fiber
- 3 g sugar
- 16 g protein

TOTINO'S
Cheese Party Pizza

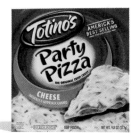

- 460 calories
- 22 g fat
- 840 mg sodium
- 2 g fiber
- 14 g protein

PRODUCE

Like most people, you probably don't spend a lot of time exploring the produce section. We've been told so much about "superfoods" like spinach, broccoli, and blueberries that most of us figure if we can eat one of those three, and maybe toss in an orange from time to time, we're good to go.

But eating only a handful of fruits and vegetables is like listening only to *The Joshua Tree*. Among the best? Sure, but there's a whole world of hard-rocking U2 hits out there, and why live without them? You might even find your most favorite song of all on an obscure early album. (I'm a fan of *Live at Red Rocks* myself.)

Same goes for fruits and vegetables. You may have even heard that certain types of produce, like celery, cucumbers, or potatoes weren't that rich in nutrients, so maybe you skip them and just concentrate on the aforementioned "superfoods." But in reality, scientists are discovering new micronutrients practically every day, and they're finding them in all sorts of produce. Chances are, we'll learn something in just the next few years that completely

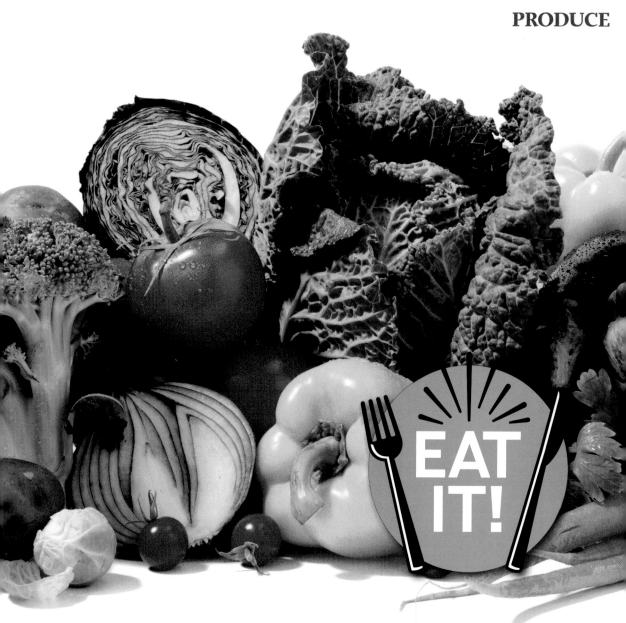

EAT
IT!

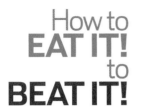

How to EAT IT! to BEAT IT!

changes the way we look at grapefruit or ginger or green beans. So don't make the mistake of limiting yourself. You could be missing the nutritional equivalent of *Achtung, Baby.*

And as you explore the produce aisle, you may want to take a look in the organic section. Many of our reliable foods are treated with pretty high levels of chemicals designed to kill bugs, mold, and more, and many absorb those chemicals into their skins and retain them. Pesticides and herbicides that have been linked to weight gain and other health issues are still being used regularly; others were banned years ago, but still linger in our soil. Of course, organic is usually more expensive, and a lot of produce that's raised conventionally is mostly pollutant free—so if you want to go organic, you need to consider only the produce highlighted in **green**.

Apples

Polyphenols in apples can regulate blood sugar and improve heart and vascular health. The fiber helps keep you satiated and decreases the amount of fat in your blood. Smaller apples pack more flavor and more nutrients.

Artichokes

High fiber and packed with antioxidants. Look for a rich green color and tightly closed leaves.

Arugula

Rich in immune-boosting, cancer-fighting glucosinolates. Look for bright green leaves, avoid it if it's started to yellow. Bigger leaf=more bitter taste.

Asparagus

High in vitamin K, which works with vitamin D to build strong bones. Also high in phytonutrients called saponins, which are anti-inflammatory and help improve blood pressure and control blood fat levels. To make asparagus last longer, trim the bottoms and stand them upright in a little water; cover with plastic and put in the fridge.

Avocados

High in heart-healthy monounsaturated fat, they're also loaded with anti-inflammatories and they help regulate blood sugar. To ripen more quickly, put them in a paper bag with an apple and leave at room temperature.

Bananas

The best source of blood-pressure-regulating potassium. Also high in fiber and B6, which protects your brain from cognitive decline.

Beets

Packed with antioxidant, anti-inflammatory, and detoxifying phytochemicals. High in folate, which reduces the amount of homocysteine in your blood, reducing your risk of heart disease.

Bell Peppers

Rich source of vitamin C and carotenoids, but go for the red, orange, or yellow varieties. Green peppers are unripened, and lower in nutrients.

Blueberries

Due to their high flavonoid content, blueberries have been shown to improve brain health, eye health, and heart function and to help regulate blood sugar. They don't store well, so if they're ripe, eat 'em. Wild blueberries, available in your freezer section, are even more powerful.

Bok Choy

Rich in cancer-fighting glucosinolates and high in immune-boosting vitamin C. Plus, it's just fun to say "bok choy."

Broccoli

High in phytonutrients, powerful cancer and inflammation fighters, and in vitamin K, which helps build strong bones.

Don't worry about the stems—most of the good stuff is in the more tender florets.

Brussels Sprouts
Very high in cancer-fighting glucosinolates. Look for smaller heads, which are sweeter, and cut an X in the bottom of the stem to reduce bitterness further.

Cabbage
Rich in immune-boosting, cancer fighting glucosinolates and high in vitamin K. Eat more cole slaw.

Cantaloupe
High in beta-carotene (thirty times more than oranges) and vitamins A and C. Research suggests it is protective against metabolic syndrome (the combination of weight gain, diabetes, and heart disease).

Carrots
Vitamin A powerhouse, chock-full of antioxidants, offering cardiovascular and cancer protection. Buy them with greens attached, to preserve freshness.

Cauliflower
High in vitamin C and fiber, it also has compounds called isothiocyanates that are shown to block the progression of some aggressive cancers. Don't store it near fruit, as it will go bad more quickly.

Celery
High in luteolin, which reduces age-related inflammation in the brain and protects against age-related memory loss. Avoid wobbly or cracked stalks.

Chard
High in vitamins K and A and metabolism-protecting magnesium. Also contains syringic acid, which can help regulate blood sugar.

Collard Greens
Vitamin K explosions, extremely efficient at shuttling fats from the body and lowering cholesterol. Look for smaller leaves, which are more tender.

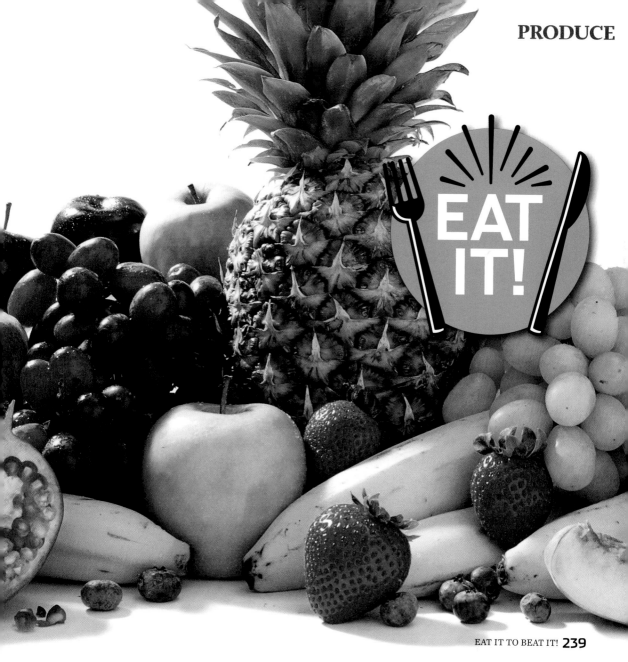

EAT
IT!

Corn

High in fiber and good for digestive health. Peel the top of the husk and press a kernel with your fingernail. If it spits at you, it's ripe.

Cucumber

Contains polyphenols called lignans that are protective against cardiovascular disease and various cancers.

Eggplant

Skin contains a compound called nasunin, which is a potent antioxidant, specifically targeting free radicals that affect the brain.

Fennel

Contains antioxidants like kaempferol, quercetin, anethole, and limonene, which give it powerful anti-inflammatory and anti-cancer properties.

Figs

High in satiating fiber—about 1½ gram in each fruit—and polyphenols, which can reduce cancer risk.

Garlic

Contains the sulfur compound allicin, which is protective against cancer, heart disease, and may even interrupt the formation of fat cells. It also wipes out *Helicobacter pylori* bacteria, which causes peptic ulcers. If it has a powdery substance on the head, it's moldy.

Ginger

Rich in antioxidants, it can reduce cholesterol levels, and ease nausea and sooth an upset stomach by breaking down fatty foods and digesting proteins.

Grapefruit

Packed with free-radical-cleansing vitamin C, has been shown to be protective against gum disease, prevent kidney stones, and protect against cancer. (May interfere with some prescription drugs.)

Grapes

Red grapes contain the potent antioxidant resveratrol, which has been linked to longevity. Grapes are also good sources of potassium.

Green Beans

High in fiber and packed with antioxidants. Use them as a snack with dip in place of chips.

Honeydew

High in heart-protecting potassium and inflammation-battling vitamin C.

Kale

Very high in vitamin K, beta carotene, and lutein; all are protective of heart health and vision health. Also, a great non-dairy source of bone-protecting calcium.

Kiwi

High in fiber and vitamin C, protects against DNA damage, macular degeneration, and heart disease.

Leeks

Contain the flavonoid kaempferol, which can protect the lining of our blood vessels from oxidative stress.

Lemons/Limes

High in phytonutrients called flavonol glycosides, which protect against cell damage, and in compounds called limonoids, which protect against various cancers.

Lettuce (Green or Romaine)

High in heart-healthy vitamin C and vitamin K, which helps blood clot properly and protects our bones.

Mangoes

High in fiber and vitamin C.

Mushrooms (Shiitake)

Filled with immune-building, cancer-protecting, cholesterol-lowering compounds like lentinan. Plus a good non-animal source of iron.

Onion
High in cancer-fighting quercetin. Also contains a peptide called GPCS that is protective against osteoporosis.

Oranges
Contains the phytonutrient herperidin, which has been shown to lower high blood pressure and cholesterol. Also high in vitamin C.

Peaches
High in fiber, vitamin A, and potassium. And an antioxidant called chlorogenic acid, which helps fight free-radical damage.

Pears
The flesh isn't particularly nutritious, but the skin contains anti-inflammatory flavonoids and anti-cancer compounds, plus lots of fiber.

Pineapple
High in vitamin C and manganese, which helps give you energy and fight infections.

Plums
Contain powerful antioxidant phenols that are particularly good at targeting free radicals that attack our brains.

Potatoes (Red)
Contain blood-pressure-lowering phytochemicals known as kukoamines that rival the amounts found in broccoli.

Raspberries
Contain an antioxidant called rheosim that increases fat cell metabolism. Also high in cancer-fighting antioxidants and belly-busting fiber. Don't wash them until right before you eat them, or they will go mushy.

Spinach
Molecules called glycoglycero-lipids can help protect the lining of your digestive tract from free-radical damage.

Squash (Butternut)
Packed with immune-boosting vitamin A and starch

compounds called polysaccharides that have powerful antioxidant, anti-inflammatory, blood-sugar-regulating qualities.

Strawberries
Packed with vitamin C and anti-inflammatory phyto-nutrients like anthocyanins, ellagitannins, flavonols, terpenoids, and phenolic acids.

Sweet Potatoes
These beta-carotene super-heroes are also packed with antioxidant anthocyanin pigments, which can protect against vision loss, cancer, hypertension, and age-related mental decline. Plus, when else can you justify eating melted marshmallows?

Tomatoes
High in the cancer-fighting carotenoid lycopene. Off-season, choose Romas or cherry tomatoes.

Watermelon
High in lycopene and the amino acid citrulline, which is converted to arginine in the body, which relaxes blood vessels and improves blood flow.

Zucchini/Yellow Squash
High in fiber and vitamin C, along with free-radical-scrubbing lutein and zeaxanthin.

RICE & RICE DISHES

It started with your neighbor's first cousin. Then your former roommate's new husband was diagnosed with it. Then you read about some celebrities who came down with it. Suddenly, your uncle had it, then your dad and your sister, and now you wonder if it's got you, too.

Super-contagious zombie-apocalypse virus?

Nope. The totally not-contagious yet spreading-like-wildfire condition called gluten intolerance. With everyone from Zooey Deschanel to Chelsea Clinton to tennis star Novak Djokovic suddenly gluten-free, wheat has fallen out of favor. And since rice doesn't contain gluten—the protein found in wheat, barley, and rye—it is on the rise, both as a dish and as an ingredient in other

BOGUS LABEL ALERT! *You'll often see "autolyzed yeast extract" in rice products claiming to be "all natural" and "additive free." But this ingredient is actually a hidden source of MSG. The FDA says these products can't claim to be MSG-free, but they don't have to alert you that they contain MSG either. Other hidden MSG sources are: hydrolyzed vegetable protein, hydrolyzed yeast, yeast extract, soy extracts, and protein isolate.*

It's just rice, with a little herbal flavoring. What could possibly be wrong? Well, when it comes to the actual flavor of rice, the folks at Rice-a-Roni think you can't handle the truth, so they've added some monosodium glutamate to this box. But look further, and you'll find five additional, hidden forms of MSG. It also includes ferric orthophosphate, a pesticide used to kill slugs and snails; it was banned from use in food in Europe a few years ago. Guys, come on . . . do you really have a snail problem?

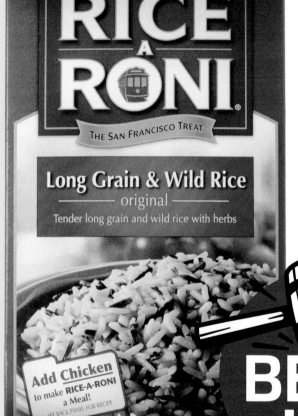

WORST "PLAIN" RICE

Rice-a-Roni Long Grain & Wild Rice
(Original, prepared)

240 Calories
6 g fat
1 g trans fat
1 g fiber
840 mg sodium

BEAT IT!

foods like bread. Which should be a good thing: In its original form, rice is a near perfect food. Key words: original form.

Unfortunately, most of the rice we consume today is white rice, meaning that the rice seeds are milled to strip them of their bran and germ—the two parts of the seed that pack most of the fiber, magnesium, potassium, and important B vitamins. Manufacturers are required by law in the United States to add back vitamins B1, B3, and iron to white rice via a process called enrichment, but that fat-fighting fiber will never come back. (Oh, and the "enrichment" vitamins will partially boil off when you cook the rice.) And that's before the food gurus really begin to have their wicked way with this wonder food. . . .

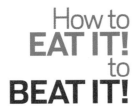

If the answer were simply to order brown rice and be done with it, we'd all be fine. One cup of brown rice delivers an entire day's worth of whole grains—48 grams' worth. But food growers and manufacturers have a few additional tricks up their sleeves that consumers need to know about.

THE RICE RULES

CHOOSE RICE THAT'S GONE HOLLYWOOD. Some rice lists its state and/or country of origin. If you can find it, look for rice grown in California. Most of the rice from the South is grown on land that used to grow cotton, where arsenic-containing pesticides were used for decades; the FDA released a 2012 study showing higher levels of arsenic in rice from these regions. And rice from Asia and Europe can have significant lead content. That makes Cali our clean-eating winner.

A gluten-free rice bowl, what could be healthier, right? Wrong. This rice bowl has as many carbs as ten Krispy Kreme donuts, and as much sodium as two large bags of Cape Cod potato chips. All rice is "gluten free" (nice head fake, P.F.), but with this dish, your own glutes will soon be charged for extra carry-on baggage.

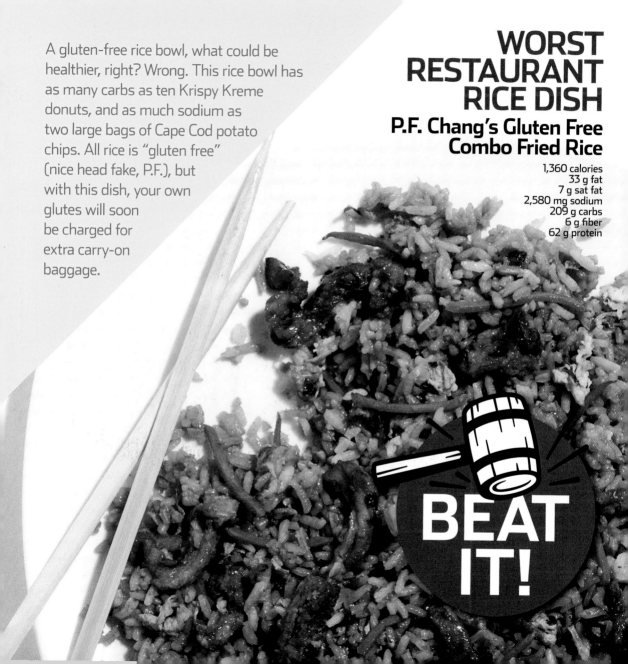

WORST RESTAURANT RICE DISH

P.F. Chang's Gluten Free Combo Fried Rice

1,360 calories
33 g fat
7 g sat fat
2,580 mg sodium
209 g carbs
6 g fiber
62 g protein

BEAT IT!

BATHE YOUR RICE. Rinsing the rice before you cook it and cooking it in a lot of water (about a 6-to-1 ratio) will cut contaminants like arsenic by about 30 percent. You just need to drain it afterward like you would pasta.

AVOID HIDDEN MSG. Look out for the words "autolyzed yeast extract," "hydrolyzed vegetable protein," "hydrolyzed yeast," "yeast extract," "soy extracts," and "protein isolate." These ingredients naturally contain MSG.

BEWARE THE BOX. Generally these boxed rice concoctions contain a lot of salt and added ingredients that you don't want on your plate, like MSG, trans fats, and coloring.

GO LONG. Choose a long-grain rice like basmati, Carolina, jasmine, or Texmati. There's a bit more fiber, so it'll keep you satiated a bit longer than short grain or white rice.

ACT SPUDLY. Unless you really like rice, and you're eating sushi, or a burrito, or possibly some risotto with a nice piece of osso buco on top, don't order rice at a restaurant. You're adding about 200 to 300 calories of fast-absorbing carbs to your meal along with whatever flavor enhancers (read MSG) the restaurant deems fit for consumption. In general, you're better off with the baked potato.

THE RICE ADVANTAGE

Lose Weight

Rice (both white and brown) is famous for making people feel fuller faster, allowing them to consume fewer calories. Whole grains are incredibly important to a healthy diet, and brown rice is widely available. If you eat primarily white rice, consider making the switch to brown to get that much more of a nutritional punch. A study in the *American Journal of Clinical Nutrition* found that women who eat more whole grains, like brown rice, are 49 percent less likely to gain weight than people who eat more refined grains. A 2009 study from the *Journal of the American Dietetic Association* found that rice-eaters make healthier choices overall.

Beat Diabetes

Switching to brown rice may also prevent diabetes. A study from researchers at the Harvard Department of Nutrition found that people who ate two servings of brown rice per week had a much lower risk of developing type 2 diabetes. They estimated that switching from white rice to brown rice lowered diabetes risk by 16 percent.

There are **100,000 varieties of rice** conserved in the International Rice Genebank in the Philippines.

and none of them are named "A-RONI"

BEST RESTAURANT RICE DISH

Red Lobster Wild Rice Pilaf

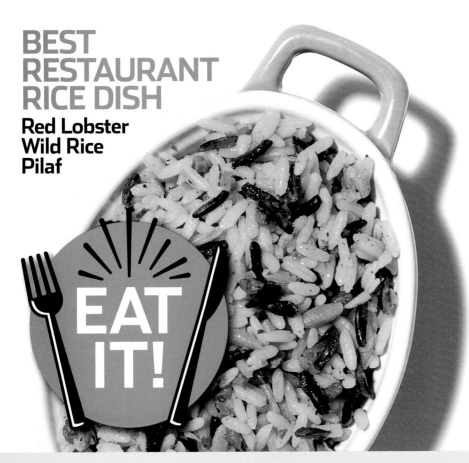

EAT IT!

MOE'S SOUTHWEST GRILL
Side of rice
- 110 calories
- 0 fat
- 135 mg sodium
- 3 g protein

CHIPOTLE MEXICAN GRILL
Side of rice
- 170 calories
- 4 g fat
- 200 mg sodium
- 2.5 g protein

POPEYES
Red Beans & Rice
- 230 calories
- 14 g fat
- 580 mg sodium
- 5 g fiber
- 0 g sugar
- 7 g protein

Red Lobster keeps it simple with one of the lowest-calorie rice dishes you'll find in any restaurant.

180 Calories
3 g fat
650 mg sodium
4 g protein

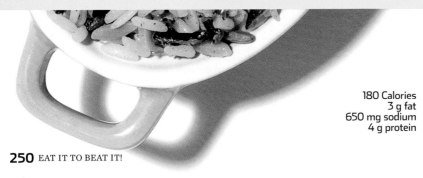

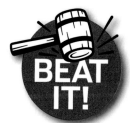

BEAT IT!

P.F. CHANG'S
Pork Fried Rice

1,370 calories
41 g fat
2,130 mg sodium
5 g fiber
51 g protein

All P.F. Chang's fried rice meals have over 1,000 calories and over 2,000 mg sodium.

PANDA EXPRESS
Steamed Brown Rice

420 calories
4 g fat
15 mg sodium
4 g fiber
1 g sugar
9 g protein

TGI FRIDAY'S
Jasmine Rice Pilaf

420 calories
11 g fat
470 g sodium
5 g fiber
7 g protein

THE CHEESECAKE FACTORY
Steamed White Rice

310 calories
0 sodium
0 fiber
0 sugar
0 protein

PLAIN GRAIN BRAIN DRAIN

Not only are most prepackaged rice dishes—Zatarian's, Near East, Uncle Ben's, Goya—built from nutrient-deprived white rice, but most are packed with MSG and plenty of other things the Buddha never ate. You'll save money—and lots of worry—by skipping the prepackaged dishes and cooking this, in the same amount of time.

Rice-a-Phonie

Here's a great way to cut down on both your food bill and your exposure to MSG, sodium, and pesticides: Make this super-fast, super-easy at-home version of your favorite San Francisco treat. You'll get two-thirds less fat and one-twelfth less sodium than the boxed version.

▼

Heat the butter in a pot or large saucepan over medium heat. Sweat the onions and garlic until soft and translucent, about 5 minutes. Stir in the rice, cook for a few minutes until lightly toasted, then add the broth and the bay leaf, plus a pinch or two of salt. Bring to a simmer, then turn the heat to low, cover, and cook until the liquid has been absorbed and the rice is tender, about 17 to 20 minutes. Remove the lid and fluff with a fork before serving.

MAKES 4 SERVINGS

1 Tbsp butter

¼ cup minced onion

1 clove garlic, minced

1 cup long-grain brown rice

1 ½ cups low-sodium chicken broth

1 bay leaf

Salt to taste

221 calories
5 g fat
2 g sat fat
56 mg sodium
1 g sugar
6 g protein
2 g fiber

BEST SUPERMARKET RICE

Lundberg Organic White Basmati

CALIFORNIA WHITE BASMATI RICE

This long-grain organic California rice tested the lowest for arsenic and contains 160 calories, 3 g protein, 1 g fiber, and 34 g of carbohydrates (1.3 to 1.6 micrograms of inorganic arsenic per serving).

EAT IT!

TRADER JOE'S
White Basmati

150 calories
0 fiber
3 g protein
2.5 to 2.9 micrograms of inorganic arsenic per serving

CASBAH
Saffroned Jasmine Rice

170 calories
0 fiber
4 g protein

ZATARAIN'S
Big Easy Garden Vegetable Brown Rice

210 calories
2.5 g fat
580 mg sodium
2 g fiber
5 g protein

While most boxed rice dishes are loaded with things we can't pronounce, all 17 of the ingredients on this box are four syllables or fewer.

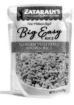

UNCLE BEN'S
Original Enriched Parboiled Long Grain Rice

170 calories
0 fiber
4 g protein
5.9 to 6.3 micrograms of inorganic arsenic per serving

365 EVERYDAY VALUE
Long Grain Brown Rice

170 calories
1.5 g fat
2 g fiber
4 g protein
7.4 to 8.4 micrograms of inorganic arsenic per serving

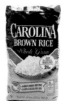

CAROLINA
Whole Grain Brown

150 calories
1 g fat
1 g fiber
3 g protein
6.4 to 8.7 micrograms of inorganic arsenic per serving

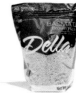

DELLA
Basmati Brown

160 calories
1 g fat
1 g fiber
3 g protein
5.9 to 9.4 micrograms of inorganic arsenic per serving

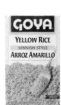

GOYA
Yellow Rice

170 calories
0 fat
546 mg sodium
1 g fiber
0 g sugar
4 g protein

ZATARAIN'S
Big Easy Dirty Rice

230 calories
3 g fat
580 mg sodium
1 g fiber
0 g sugar
5 g protein

BEAT IT!

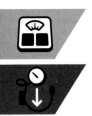

SALAD/SALAD BAR

Eating a salad is a lot like going to the gym: You feel better about yourself after you've done it, but finding the motivation to make it happen is a challenge. And unlike the gym, there are no hot, Spandexed personal trainers to flirt with at the salad bar.

But while going to the gym is always a good idea, ordering the salad, surprisingly, isn't. Eager to capitalize on our inner battle between good and evil, between our desire to be fit and healthy and our other desire to wrap ourselves in raw bacon and jump into a vat of melted cheese, some food marketers have tried to give us both at the same time—salads that make us feel like we're eating well, while at the same time giving our tastebuds a hot-oil treatment.

So be selective the next time you venture into the verdant jungle of the salad menu, or you might find you're better off with a cheeseburger.

That's as many calories as 6 Original Klondike Bars . . . in a salad.

WORST SALAD
IHOP Chicken and Spinach Salad

1,560 calories
112 g fat
30 g sat fat
2,660 mg sodium
7 g fiber
13 g sugar
67 g protein

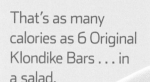

BOGUS LABEL ALERT!

Something missing in your calorie counts? Make sure that the calorie information listed for your salad includes the dressing, which can add a lot of calories and fat. Carl's Jr.'s Crispy Chicken Salad says it's 350 calories with 16 g of fat, but that's butt naked. When you add some Blue Cheese Dressing on there it becomes a 670-calorie whopper with 50 g of fat.

BEAT IT!

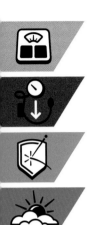

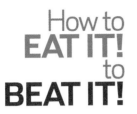

How to EAT IT! to BEAT IT!

Building a healthy salad is like winning a paintball fight: You want to spread as many bright colors around as you can. Bright colors are nature's way of signaling high-nutrient content. Skip the iceberg and load your plate with dark greens like romaine, spinach, arugula, and radicchio. Then cover the greens with tomatoes, carrots, broccoli, cucumbers, bell peppers, radishes, cantaloupe, watermelon, grapes, raisins, strawberries. Each color signifies its own unique combination of nutrients, so the more colors you have, the better.

THE SALAD BAR RULES

DRESS RIGHT. Choosing a non-fat salad dressing might give you fewer calories, but you'll miss out on some of the powerful fat-soluble disease-fighting compounds in fresh fruits and vegetables. One recent study found that dressings with monounsaturated fats (canola or olive oil-based dressings) improve the absorption of fat-soluble carotenoids, like lutein, lycopene, beta-carotene, and zeaxanthin, which are associated with a reduced risk of cancer, cardiovascular disease, obesity, diabetes, and basically every other major chronic disease.

PICK POTENT PROTEIN. When in doubt, choose beans and chickpeas. They'll give you a fiber boost as well as healthy protein. If you want some meat, go for grilled (not fried) chicken or beef. Nuts and seeds are also a great choice.

AND SKIP EVERYTHING ELSE. When it comes to bacon bits, crunchy noodles, cheese, oily croutons, mayo-soaked potato and macaroni salads, and the odd Jello offering (why is that there?) just say no. If you focus on multicolored vegetables and avoid anything that's not of this earth, you'll be fine.

THE SALAD ADVANTAGE

Lose Weight

Eating a salad before your main meal can help you consume 12 percent fewer calories, according to a study in the *Journal of the American Dietetic Association*.

Lower Blood Pressure

Boosting your potassium intake can help lower blood pressure by up to 10 percent. Best sources: bananas, avocados, white beans, spinach, dried apricots, kale.

Improve Mood

Folate, a B vitamin found in leafy greens like spinach, kale, and romaine, as well as in beans and lentils, has been shown to improve patients' response to antidepressant drugs.

Boost Immunity

Green vegetables are the source of a chemical signal that is important to a fully-functioning immune system. They help ensure that immune cells in the gut and the skin (known as intra-epithelial lymphocytes) function properly.

CAESAR SEIZURE

According to researchers at Duke University, when people spy a salad option at a restaurant, they are more likely to go to another part of the menu and order something especially unhealthy. They call the phenomenon "vicarious goal fulfillment." Just because you considered the salad option, you unconsciously feel like you have met a goal, and reward yourself with something bad for you. So don't do that, okay?

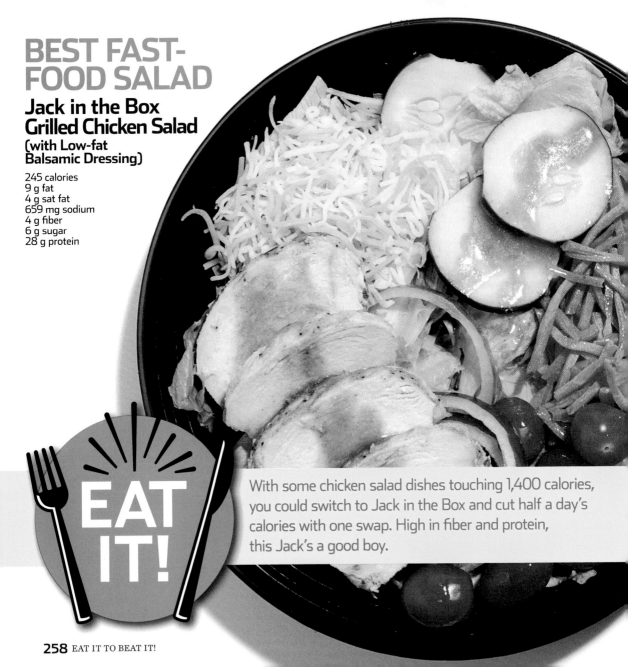

BEST FAST-FOOD SALAD

Jack in the Box Grilled Chicken Salad
(with Low-fat Balsamic Dressing)

245 calories
9 g fat
4 g sat fat
659 mg sodium
4 g fiber
6 g sugar
28 g protein

EAT IT!

With some chicken salad dishes touching 1,400 calories, you could switch to Jack in the Box and cut half a day's calories with one swap. High in fiber and protein, this Jack's a good boy.

CARL'S JR.
Grilled Chicken Salad (with Low-Fat Balsamic Vinaigrette Dressing)

- 315 calories
- 17.5 g fat
- 4.5 g sat fat
- 1,330 mg sodium
- 2 g fiber
- 10 g sugar
- 17 g protein

MCDONALD'S
Premium Southwest Salad with Grilled Chicken

- 290 calories
- 8 g fat
- 2.5 g sat fat
- 650 mg sodium
- 7 g fiber
- 11 g sugar
- 27 g protein

AU BON PAIN
Southwest Chicken Salad

- 350 calories
- 11 g fat
- 1.5 g sat fat
- 390 mg sodium
- 12 g fiber
- 9 g sugar
- 24 g protein

QUIZNOS
Small Harvest Chicken Salad

- 300 calories
- 19 g fat
- 4.5 g sat fat
- 480 mg sodium
- 2 g fiber
- 19 g sugar
- 9 g protein

IHOP
Crispy Chicken Salad with Fried Chicken

- 1,400 calories
- 88 g fat
- 26 g sat fat
- 2,770 mg sodium
- 9 g fiber
- 28 g sugar
- 66 g protein

APPLEBEE'S
Oriental Chicken Salad (Regular)

- 1,390 calories
- 98 g fat
- 15 g sat fat
- 1,600 mg sodium
- 11 g fiber
- 39 g protein

TGI FRIDAYS
Pecan-Crusted Chicken Salad

- 1,380 calories
- 102 g fat
- 21 g sat fat
- 2,030 mg sodium
- 11 g fiber
- 39 g protein

CALIFORNIA PIZZA KITCHEN
Moroccan Spiced Chicken Salad

- 1,370 calories
- 82 g fat
- 12 g sat fat
- 1,040 mg sodium
- 78 g sugar
- 23 g fiber
- 43 g protein

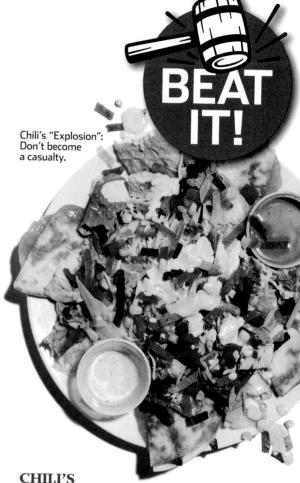

Chili's "Explosion": Don't become a casualty.

CHILI'S
Boneless Buffalo Chicken Salad

- 1,030 calories
- 67 g fat
- 15 g sat fat
- 4,720 mg sodium
- 7 g fiber
- 9 g sugar
- 51 g protein

Quesadilla Explosion Salad

- 1,430 calories
- 96 g fat
- 28 g sat fat
- 3,090 mg sodium
- 9 g fiber
- 14 g sugar
- 63 g protein

SALAD DRESSINGS

According to a Purdue University study , you want your salad dressing to have some fat in it so that the carotenoids (those magic molecules that protect you from chronic diseases like cancer and heart disease) found in vegetables are better absorbed in your body. Their study found that monounsaturated fats are better at this than polyunsaturated and saturated fats, so look for dressings that contain anywhere from 3 to 20 g of fat from olive oil or canola oil, not soybean oil.

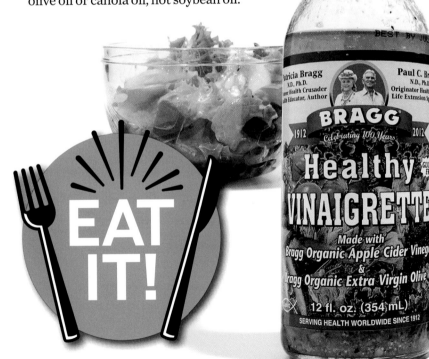

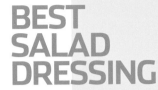

BEST SALAD DRESSING

Bragg Healthy Organic Vinaigrette

150 calories
15 g fat
2 g sat fat
120 mg sodium
0 g fiber
2 g sugar
0 g protein
2 tbsp

Contains organic extra virgin first-pressed olive oil, organic apple cider vinegar, liquid aminos, raw honey, garlic, onion, and red bell pepper flakes . . . Can you say "superfood?"

ANNIE'S

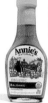

Naturals Dressing Balsamic Vinaigrette

100 calories
10 g fat
1 g sat fat
55 mg sodium
2 g sugar
1 g protein
2 tbsp

NEWMAN'S OWN

Salad Dressing Olive Oil & Vinegar All Natural

150 calories
16 g fat
2.5 g sat fat
150 mg sodium
0 g fiber
1 g sugar
1 g protein
2 tbsp

BRIANNAS

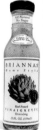

Home Style Salad Dressing Real French Vinaigrette

130 calories
14 g fat
1 g sat fat
260 mg sodium
0 g fiber
0 g sugar
0 g protein
2 tbsp

HIDDEN VALLEY

Dressing Original Ranch

140 calories
14 g fat
2.5 g sat fat
260 mg sodium
1 g sugar
1 g protein

Soybean oil is the first ingredient, and monosodium glutamate (MSG) is nestled in the ingredient list right next to artificial flavors.

WISH-BONE

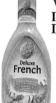

Deluxe French Dressing

120 calories
11 g fat
1.5 g sat fat
170 mg sodium
0 g fiber
5 g sugar
0 protein

Soybean oil, propylene glycol (antifreeze)

KRAFT

Classic Ranch Anytime Dressing

110 calories
11 g fat
1.5 g sat fat
300 mg sodium
0 g fiber
1 g sugar
0 g protein

Soybean oil, MSG

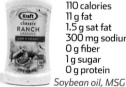

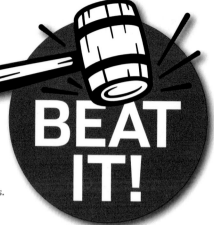

BEAT IT!

MARIE'S DRESSING

Chunky Blue Cheese

160 calories
17 g fat
3.5 g sat fat
170 mg sodium
0 g fiber
0 g sugar
1 g protein

KEN'S STEAK HOUSE DRESSING

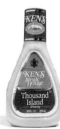

Thousand Island

140 calories
13 g fat
2 g sat fat
300 mg sodium
0 g fiber
3 g sugar
0 g protein

Soybean oil, high fructose corn syrup, propylene glycol (antifreeze)

SANDWICHES

They say a sandwich always tastes better when someone else makes it, but your tastes might change once you realize what they've been feeding you all these years.

The complexity of a sandwich makes it a great place to hide a lot of evils. A commercially made sandwich is like a new bill passed by Congress. It might have a really great title—"The Meatballs & Mozzarella Hot Pocket Act of 2014"—but it can be loaded with lots of unnecessary fat, political sweeteners, and corrupted pork. For example, the above-mentioned Hot Pocket lists 112 ingredients, many of which exceed five syllables, including something called L-cysteine hydrochloride. The cheapest and most common source of L-cysteine, a dough conditioner, is human hair, although duck feathers are also commonly used.

Lunch is the part of the day when the average American diet can often go haywire. Breakfast is controllable and pretty easy to figure out, and dinner, especially if you're at home, is still a task that one can manage. But the noon hour is a time for fast food, business lunches, vending machines, and anything else that can be scarfed down in enough time to still run a few errands before we need to rush back to work and reapply our nose to the grindstone.

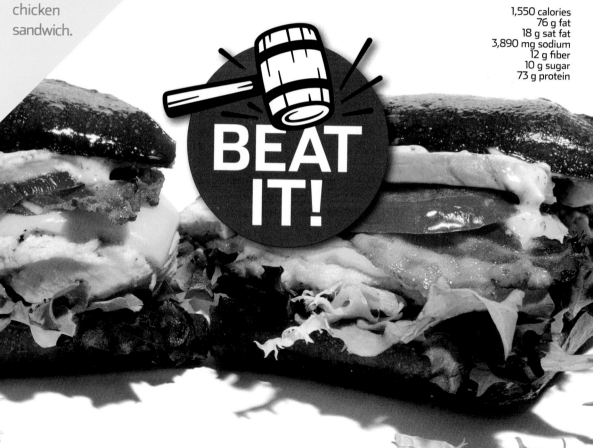

It would take 35 servings of Tostitos Multigrain Tortilla Chips—or about 283 chips—to equal the amount of sodium in this chicken sandwich.

WORST RESTAURANT SANDWICH

Chili's Bacon Avocado Chicken Sandwich

1,550 calories
76 g fat
18 g sat fat
3,890 mg sodium
12 g fiber
10 g sugar
73 g protein

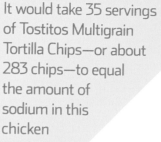

BEAT IT!

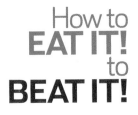

How to
EAT IT!
to
BEAT IT!

The two great advantages of the sandwich—portability and convenience—are the two biggest enemies to your weight-management plan. Most sandwiches are eaten with one hand while the other hand types, holds a phone, or steers a wheel. And that means we tend to scarf them down faster and more mindlessly than we would food eaten with a fork. As a result, we can often consume more calories in sandwich form than we can from other foods.

THE SANDWICH RULES

UNWRAP IT. Somehow wraps became synonymous with health food, and that is far from the truth. Those flat, round flour tortilla shells can pack 300 calories before you even fill them, and a lot of them are loaded with trans fats and other oils.

HOT MEANS HEAVY. Hot sandwiches usually have more calories than cold sandwiches (meatball subs and pulled pork are some of the highest calorie sandwiches out there).

WHEN IN DOUBT . . . BLT. The bacon, lettuce, tomato sandwich is a good standby burst of protein and fiber that shouldn't cost you too many calories, even with a little mayo.

STRIKE OUT THE BATTER. If the meat in your sandwich was battered and fried, you can count on it costing you calories and fat, often trans fats. Look for grilled sandwiches instead.

Despite terms like "reduced sugar" and "whole wheat" on the label, there's high fructose corn syrup, hydrogenated oil, and azodicarbon-amide, a foaming agent used in plastics, in this Smucker's sandwich. A home-made sandwich on whole wheat would double the fiber and protein content.

WORST SUPERMARKET SANDWICH

Smucker's Uncrustables Reduced Sugar Peanut Butter & Grape Spread Sandwiches on Whole Wheat

190 calories
9 g fat
2 g sat fat
170 mg sodium
3 g fiber
6 g sugar
7 g protein

BEAT IT!

TYSON
Buffalo Mini Grilled Chicken Sandwiches

300 calories
8 g fat
2 g sat fat
810 mg sodium
1 g fiber
6 g sugar
22 g protein

NEW!

High sodium, contains MSG

LEAN POCKETS
Sandwiches, Pretzel Bread, Chicken Jalapeno Cheddar

270 calories
8 g fat
3.5 g sat fat
700 mg sodium
2 g fiber
2 g sugar
13 g protein

Chicken is mixed with isolated soy protein and chicken flavor, contains MSG (torula yeast), wood pulp (methylcellulose), trans fats (partially hydrogenated soybean oil and partially hydrogenated vegetable oil).

HOT POCKETS
Meatballs & Mozzarella Sandwiches

330 calories
15 g fat
6 g sat fat
610 mg sodium
2 g fiber
4 g sugar
10 g protein

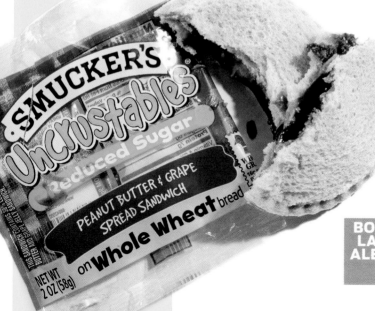

BOGUS LABEL ALERT! *Hot Pockets "Italian Style Meatballs" are made from a mixture of pork, water, textured vegetable protein, and caramel coloring. Grandma-ma, you make-a the meatballs so synthetico!*

BEST RESTAURANT SANDWICH

Subway Roast Beef Sandwich

290 calories
4.5 g fat
1.5 g sat fat
680 mg sodium
5 g fiber
7 g sugar
17 g protein

AU BON PAIN
Black Angus Roast Beef and Cheddar Sandwich

510 calories
18 g fat
8 g sat fat
1,730 mg sodium
3 g fiber
4 g sugar
33 g protein

CARL'S JR.
Charbroiled BBQ Chicken Sandwich

390 calories
7 g fat
1.5 g sat fat
990 mg sodium
3 g fiber
13 g sugar
30 g protein

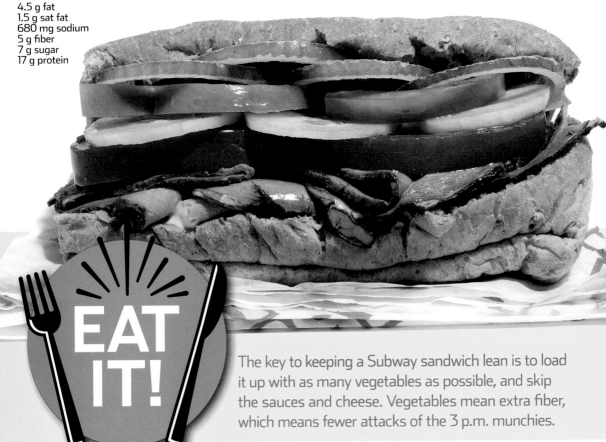

EAT IT!

The key to keeping a Subway sandwich lean is to load it up with as many vegetables as possible, and skip the sauces and cheese. Vegetables mean extra fiber, which means fewer attacks of the 3 p.m. munchies.

COSI

Fire Roasted Veggie Sandwich

373 calories
10 g fat
3 g sat fat
357 mg sodium
5 g fiber
2 g sugar
17 g protein

Hummus & Veggie Sandwich

417 calories
7 g fat
0 sat fat
552 mg sodium
7 g fiber
5 g sugar
17 g protein

PANERA BREAD

Roasted Turkey & Avocado BLT on Sourdough

510 calories
22 g fat
3.5 g sat fat
940 mg sodium
6 g fiber
2 g sugar
32 g protein

TIM HORTON'S

Turkey Bacon Club Sandwich

370 calories
7g fat
2 g sat fat
1,320 mg sodium
5 g fiber
7 g sugar
21 g protein

APPLEBEE'S

Oriental Chicken Rollup

1,190 calories
62 g fat
11 g sat fat
3,290 mg sodium
6 g fiber
35 g protein

BLIMPIE'S

Chicken Cheddar Bacon Ranch

1,200 calories
59 g fat
19 g sat fat
3,240 mg sodium
6 g fiber
17 g sugar
77 g protein

OUTBACK

Prime Rib Dip Sandwich

1,008 calories
6 g sat fat
2,350 mg sodium
62 g carbs

TGI FRIDAY'S

Jack Daniel's Chicken Sandwich

1,140 calories
58 g fat
18 g sat fat
3,140 mg sodium
4 g fiber
51 g protein

FRIENDLY'S

Honey BBQ Chicken Supermelt

1,500 calories
78 g fat
24 g sat fat
2,410 mg sodium
7 g fiber
41 g sugar
48 g protein

CHEESECAKE FACTORY

BBQ pulled Pork Sandwich

1,438 calories
25 g sat fat
2,608 mg sodium
107 g carbs

Spicy Crispy Chicken sandwich
(with chipotle mayo)

1,384 calories
22 g sat fat
2,174 mg sodium
86 g carbs

BOB EVANS

Smokehouse Fried Chicken Sandwich

1,027 calories
57 g fat
19 g sat fat
2,833 mg sodium
4 g fiber
7 g sugar
48 g protein

UNO CHICAGO GRILL

Crunchy Chicken Wrap

1,030 calories
59 g fat
17 g sat fat
2,180 mg sodium
12 g fiber
28 g sugar
61 g protein

OLIVE GARDEN

Italian Meatball Sandwich

1,050 calories
58 g fat
27 g sat fat
2,050 mg sodium
9 g fiber
54 g protein

RUBY TUESDAY'S

Chicken BLT

1,251 calories
55 g fat
3,042 mg sodium
11 g fiber
46 g protein

CALIFORNIA PIZZA KITCHEN

Italian Deli Sandwich
(with herb cheese)

1,260 calories
81 g fat
23 g sat fat
2,862 mg sodium
14 g sugar
4 g fiber
47 g protein

QUIZNOS

Chicken Carbonara
(large)

1,370 calories
68 g fat
29 g sat fat
3,110 mg sodium
4 g fiber
13 g sugar
82 g protein

IHOP

Chicken Clubhouse Super Stacker

1,210 calories
83 g fat
31 g sat fat
2,750 mg sodium
3 g fiber
12 g sugar
57 g protein

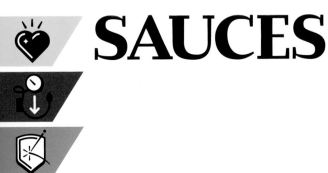

SAUCES

Every classic gangster movie, whether it stars Al Pacino or Chow Yun-Fat, is going to eventually involve a great gun battle inside an ethnic restaurant. Is it because Mafia wives are lousy cooks? (Of course not, I am totally certain all your wives are great cooks, Mafia guys. No need to send the horse's head.)

No, it's because great, heaping plates of noodles or rice smothered in sauce make awesome, operatic props as their about-to-be consumers suddenly plop face-first into them. But making sure you aren't the one plopping head-first into your dinner means making a few wise-guy choices.

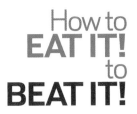

How to EAT IT! to BEAT IT!

THE SAUCE RULES

BEWARE THE WHITE STUFF. That's salt and refined sugar. For red sauces, look to stay below 400 mg of sodium and 6 grams of sugar per half-cup serving. For chili and stir-fry sauces, stay under 150 mg of sodium and 2 g sugar per tablespoon. The best Alfredo sauces max out at 600 mg sodium and 2 g sugar or less per half a cup.

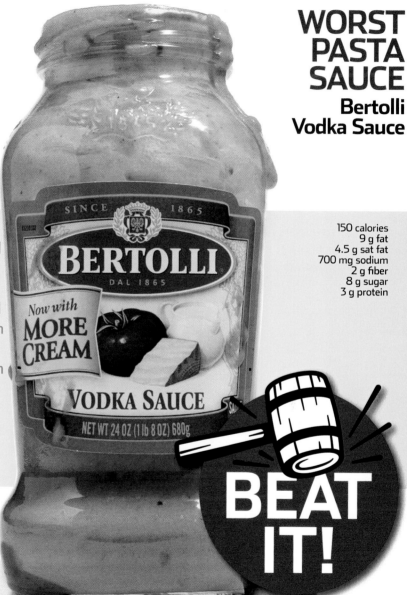

A mere half-cup serving will give you nearly a third of your daily sodium and nearly a quarter of your saturated fat intake—and you haven't even put it on the pasta, cheese, or meat yet! Add in as much sugar as 3 bowls of Kix cereal, and you might be better off skipping the sauce and going straight for the vodka.

150 calories
9 g fat
4.5 g sat fat
700 mg sodium
2 g fiber
8 g sugar
3 g protein

BERTOLLI
DAL 1865
Now with MORE CREAM
VODKA SAUCE
NET WT 24 OZ (1 lb 8 OZ) 680g

BEAT IT!

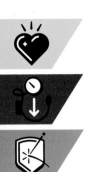

SEE RED. The health benefits of a big pasta dish are primarily found in the tomato sauce. The more your meal looks like a Quentin Tarantino movie, the better.

THE MARINARA ADVANTAGE

Boost Immunity
Research conducted on rats found that lycopene, the antioxidant that gives tomatoes its red color, was worthy of consideration as an immunity and antitumor medication. More research is needed to confirm its full effect on cancer and cancer prevention, though.

Lower Cholesterol
Researchers at Brigham and Women's Hospital and Harvard Medical School tested more than 25,000 women and found that women consuming more than ten servings of tomato-based products per week had better cholesterol numbers than those who averaged 1.5 servings per week.

Lower Blood Pressure
A study conducted by the department of health at the Iran University of Medical Sciences tested 32 type 2 diabetes patients by giving them raw tomato for eight weeks. There were significant decreases in blood pressure, which can be beneficial for reducing cardiovascular risk associated with type 2 diabetes.

BEST SAUCES

Muir Glen Organic Tomato Basil

CLASSICO
Light Creamy Alfredo

90 calories
6 g fat
4 g sat fat
600 mg sodium
0 g fiber
2 g sugar
2 g protein
½ cup

LA CHOY
Teriyaki Stir Fry Sauce & Marinade

10 calories
0 g fat
0 g sat fat
105 mg sodium
1 g sugar
0 g fiber
0 g protein
1 Tbsp

MUIR GLEN Organic

Tomato Basil
organic pasta sauce

180 calories
6 g fat
410 mg sodium

USDA ORGANIC

60 calories
1 g fat
0 g sat fat
260 mg sodium
2 g fiber
4 g sugar
2 g protein
½ cup

EAT IT!

Big food companies like to pack lots of high fructose corn syrup into places where it makes no sense, like tomato sauces. Muir Glen adds just a hint of sugar to theirs.

PREGO
Alfredo Sauce Flavored with Savory Bacon

BEAT IT!

140 calories
12 g fat
6 g sat fat
800 mg sodium
0 g fiber
2 g sugar
4 g protein
½ cup

Despite the heaping amounts of fat and sodium, the first ingredient in this food is water. It also has "enzyme modified liquid egg product" and "smoke flavoring."

AMY'S
Organic Tomato Basil

110 calories
6 g fat
1 g sat fat
580 mg sodium
6 g sugar
3 g fiber
2 g protein
½ cup

All that fat comes from olive oil, but Amy's still has twice the sodium of Muir Glen.

LA CHOY
Teriyaki Marinade and Sauce

40 calories
0 g fat
0 g sat fat
570 mg sodium
8 g sugar
0 g fiber
0g protein
1 Tbsp

Look out! Choose this product and you're getting more than five times as much salt and sugar as the same company's Teriyaki Stir Fry Sauce.

SODA, TEA, & ENERGY DRINKS

Imagine waking up every day and downing a smoothie made from 2 bowls of Corn Pops and 27 slices of Hillshire Farms pastrami. Or a frappé made from a Hebrew National hot dog and one Cold Stone Oreo Creme ice cream sandwich. Or a refreshing shake of In-N-Out Burger patty and 14 Funyuns.

A little heavy, right?

But that's what it takes to make about 465 liquid calories, which is what the average American drinks—that's right, drinks—every single day. That's an entire additional meal and about double what nutrition experts recommend. And the majority of those calories come from soft drinks—sodas, bottled iced teas, energy drinks, and the like.

The Beverage Guidance Panel, a group of Elliot Ness–like nutritionists, suggest we get no more than 250 calories a day from beverages—215 calories fewer

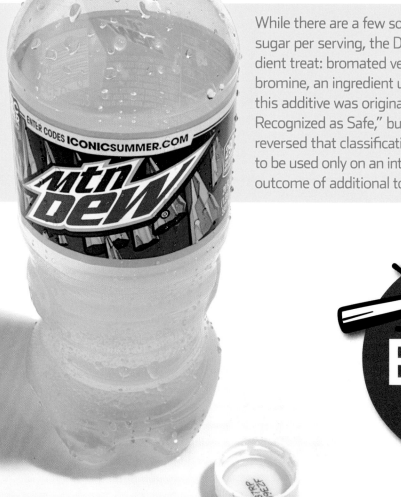

Mountain Dew
(12 oz)

170 calories
46 g sugar

While there are a few sodas that offer more sugar per serving, the Dew offers a special ingredient treat: bromated vegetable oil. Made from bromine, an ingredient used in flame retardants, this additive was originally deemed "Generally Recognized as Safe," but the FDA has since reversed that classification, and now it is allowed to be used only on an interim basis "pending the outcome of additional toxicological studies."

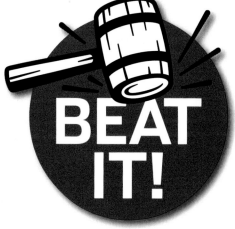

BEAT IT!

than we drink today. If we all made that simple change, and didn't alter a single thing we ate, we'd still weigh an average of 22 ½ pounds less a year from now.

In fact, liquid calories may actually cause you to gain weight faster than food calories, simply because they're absorbed faster. That means a more rapid sugar spike, and more fat storage. Here's what studies show about your risk of weight gain based on your daily soda intake.

½ can = 26 percent increased risk of being overweight or obese
½ to 1 can = 30.4 percent increased risk
1 to 2 cans = 32.8 percent increased risk
More than 2 cans = 47.2 percent increased risk

And a recent study published by the European Association for the Study of Diabetes shows that drinking just one 12-ounce sugar-sweetened soda a day can increase your risk of type 2 diabetes by 22 percent.

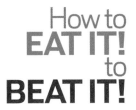

How to
EAT IT!
to
BEAT IT!

If you've ever wandered into an antiques shop on some rural Midwestern road and seen a collection of early twentieth-century Coke bottles on display, you've probably thought, "Wow, those are small." Soda was originally sold in 6-ounce bottles, and was considered a treat. Nowadays, 16-ounce bottles of sugar accompany every meal. And that's the crux of the problem.

BOGUS LABEL ALERT! *Lipton claims that a serving of their PureLeaf Lemon Iced Tea has 18 g of sugar. But each bottle is 2.5 servings—which only makes sense if the cast of* Two and a Half Men *is drinking it. If you are not a fictional sitcom character, you're more likely to drink the whole bottle and get 45 g of sugar and 175 calories.*

WORST BOTTLED TEA

Gold Peak Sweet Iced Tea
(18.5 oz)

190 calories
50 g sugar

Props to Gold Peak for admitting that a serving size is one bottle of tea. But that's where the props end, because 17 Starburst Fruit Chews' worth of sugar is way too much for one little drink.

WORST ENERGY DRINK

Rockstar Punched Energy/Punch Fruit Punch Flavor Energy
(16 oz)

260 calories
64 g sugar

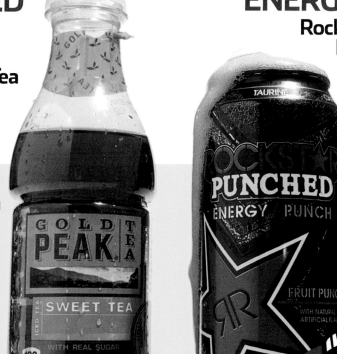

BOGUS LABEL ALERT! *"Negative Calorie Drink." Celsius Energy Drinks are marketed as "the world's first negative calorie drink," because, according to the company, their proprietary blend of ingredients raises body heat. But then they go on to say that Celsius energy drinks alone "do not produce weight loss in the absence of a healthy diet and exercise." Which is like saying you can eat "negative calorie pasta," as long as you run a marathon the next day.*

BEAT IT!

THE SOFT DRINK RULES

TREAT SODA LIKE CANDY. A 16-ounce bottle of Coke or Pepsi is the sugar equivalent of 65 Jelly Bellys, or more than two whole packages of Peanut M&M'S. A 16-ounce resealable bottle should last you three days—not one meal.

DON'T "DIET" WITH DIET. Drinking diet soda has been linked to weight gain, heart disease, diabetes, and high blood pressure. While scientists aren't sure why zero-calorie sodas cause weight gain, research suggests that when you eat or drink something sweet and your body doesn't get the calories and sugar it is expecting, your body gets confused and that confusion can lead to overeating, and blood sugar spikes that rival sugary drinks.

BEWARE TRENDY INGREDIENTS. Some energy drinks claim they can help you lose weight and burn fat. They contain an

WHAT'S IN THERE?

Soda

8.9 parts carbonated water
0.89 parts sweetener
0.1 part citric acid
0.033 parts caramel color
0.033 parts flavoring
0.033 parts caffeine

Energy Drink

8.45 parts carbonated water
1.23 parts sweetener
0.15 parts "special energy formula" (usually caffeine, taurine, guarana, etc.)
0.1 part citric acid
0.03 parts B vitamins
0.03 parts natural and artificial flavors

Bottled Tea

8.87 parts water
0.97 parts sweetener
0.027 parts tea
0.03 parts citric acid
03 parts natural flavors
0.03 parts caffeine

ingredient called DMAA (dimethylamylamine, mehtylhexanamine, or geranium extract). It's often referred to as a "natural" stimulant but can lead to serious cardiovascular problems.

DON'T GET OVERSERVED. Read the nutrition panel on the back of many drinks and you'll find 2, 2.5, even 4 servings in one little bottle. This is how they hide how much sugar you're really getting.

BREW AWAY TROUBLE

Tea, especially green tea, is packed with polyphenols, an antioxidant with enormous health benefits. But a study from the American Chemical Society found that in some cases you'd have to drink 20 bottles of prepackaged tea to get the polyphenols contained in one cup of home-brewed tea. Here's what you'd be missing.

Some research suggests drinking green tea can reduce heart attack risk, and one recent study found that people who drank two to three cups of green tea daily had a 14 percent lower risk of stroke compared to those who rarely drank it.

A study of men in China who drink black tea found that it could help fight diabetes because it slows glucose absorption.

Green tea has been found to reduce inflammation and inhibit prostate cancer growth. Another study found that women who drink green tea have a lower risk of developing GI cancers.

A flavonoid in green tea called gallated catechins has been shown to slow weight gain because it slows the absorption of fat and speeds the body's ability to use fat.

One recent study found that older adults who drank green tea daily showed improved memory ability; another study showed that extracts of green tea interfered with the creation of the amyloid plaques associated with Alzheimer's.

BEST DRINKS

BEST TEA:
Inko's Hint O'Mint White Iced Tea Unsweetened
0 calories
0 sugar

BEST ENERGY DRINK:
GT'S Synergy Gingerberry Kombucha
70 calories
8 g sugar

BEST SODA:
GuS Grown-Up Soda, Extra Dry Ginger Ale
90 calories
22 g sugar

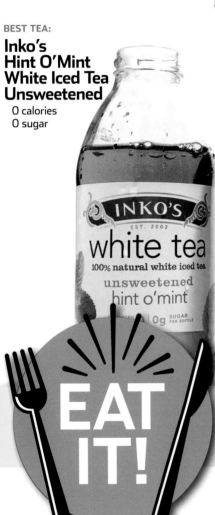

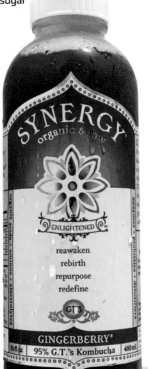

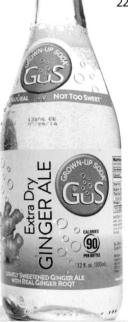

EAT IT!

GT's is the best fermented beverage on the market. It's sweet, but doesn't contain too much sugar; you'll get a great energy boost from the organic, raw fermented kombucha tea (and there's a little alcohol in there, too, so it's a great beer replacement).

SODA:

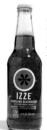

IZZE
Sparkling Blackberry
130 calories
29 g sugar

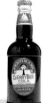

FENTIMANS
Cherry Tree Cola
(9.3 oz)
130 calories
32 g sugar

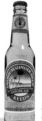

REEDS
Premium Ginger Brew
(12 oz)
145 calories
37.4 g sugar

Yes, it has a lot of sugar in it but it also has real ginger root, which can help with an upset stomach, and it makes an amazing cocktail mixer.

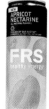

TEA:

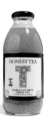

HONEST TEA
Moroccan Mint Green Tea Organic
(16 oz)
34 calories
10 g sugar

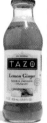

TAZO
Lemon Ginger Herbal Infusion
(13.8 oz)
70 calories
17 g sugar

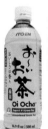

ITO EN
Oi Ocha Green Tea
(16.9 oz)
0 calories
0 sugar

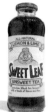

SWEET LEAF
Lemon Lime Unsweet Tea
0 calories
0 sugar

ENERGY DRINK:

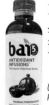

BAI
Antioxidant Infusion Pomegranate
5 calories
1 g sugar
(121 mg caffeine per 12 oz)

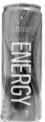

STEAZ
Energy Zero Calorie Berry
0 calories
0 sugar
(108 mg caffeine per 12 oz)

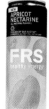

WILD BERRY
FRS Healthy Energy
90 calories
19 g sugar
(17 mg caffeine per 12 oz)

TROPICANA
Twister Soda Orange
190 calories
52 g sugar

CRUSH
Lime Soda
190 calories
50 g sugar

TROPICANA
Twister Soda Grape
190 calories
50 g sugar

MELLOW YELLOW
170 calories
47 g sugar

MOUNTAIN DEW
170 calories
46 g sugar
Brominated vegetable oil!!

A&W
Cream Soda
170 calories
45 g sugar

Root Beer
170 calories
45 g sugar

BARQ'S
Root Beer
150 calories
45 g sugar

HIRES
Root Beer
170 calories
44 g sugar

FANTA
Orange
160 calories
44 g sugar
Bromated vegetable oil!!

SUNKIST
177 calories
43 g sugar

CRUSH
Orange Soda
160 calories
43 g sugar

12 OZ MUG
Root beer
160 calories
43 g sugar

RC COLA
160 calories
42 g sugar

PEPSI
Wild Cherry
160 calories
42 g sugar

CHERRY COKE
150 calories
42 g sugar

COCA-COLA
Vanilla
150 calories
42 g fat

PEPSI
150 calories
41 g sugar

DR. PEPPER
150 calories
40 g sugar

COKE
140 calories
39 g sugar

7UP
140 calories
38 g sugar

SPRITE
140 calories
38 g sugar

SIERRA MIST
140 calories
37 g sugar

CANADA DRY GINGER ALE
140 calories
35 g sugar

SEAGRAM'S GINGER ALE
130 calories
35 g sugar

SCHWEPPES GINGER ALE
120 calories
32 g sugar

IZZE
120 calories
29 g sugar

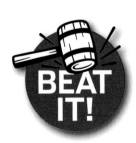

SNAPPLE
Peach Tea (16 oz)
- 160 calories
- 39 g sugar

ARIZONA
Green Tea with Ginseng and Honey (18.5 oz)
- 175 calories
- 42.5 g sugar

Iced Tea Lemon (18.5 oz)
- 225 calories
- 60 g sugar

PURE LEAF TEA
Sweet Tea (18.5 oz)
- 160 calories
- 42 g sugar

LIPTON
100% Natural Green Tea Citrus (20 oz)
- 130 calories
- 32 g sugar

Brisk Iced Tea Lemon (20 oz)
- 130 calories
- 33 g sugar

NANTUCKET NECTARS
Half & Half Half Lemonade & Half Iced Tea (16 oz)
- 180 calories
- 44 g sugar

SOBE
Energize Green Tea (20 oz)
- 200 calories
- 51 g sugar

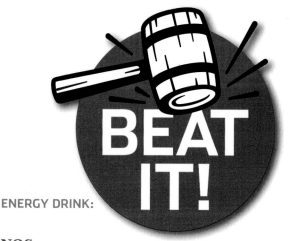

NOS
Loaded Cherry Energy Drink (16 oz)
- 210 calories
- 54 g sugar
- *(224 mg caffeine per 16 oz)*

FULL THROTTLE
Red Berry (16 oz)
- 240 calories
- 58 g sugar
- *(420 mg caffeine per 16 oz)*

ARIZONA
Caution Extreme Performance Energy Drink (16 oz)
- 240 calories
- 58 g sugar
- *(258 mg caffeine per 16 oz)*

VENOM
Energy Black Mamba (16 oz)
- 240 calories
- 53 g sugar
- *(220 mg caffeine per 16 oz)*

MONSTER
Nitrous Super Dry Energy Drink (16 oz)
- 160 calories
- 38 g sugar
- *(184 mg caffeine per 16 oz)*

RED BULL
(8.3 oz)
- 110 calories
- 27 g sugar
- *(83 mg caffeine per 8.3 oz)*

SAMBAZAN
Amazon Energy (12 oz)
- 135 calories
- 30 g sugar
- *(121 mg caffeine per 12 oz)*

AMP
Energy Boost (16 oz)
- 220 calories
- 58 g sugar
- *(142 mg caffeine per 16 oz)*

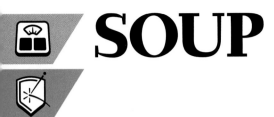

SOUP

Listen up, Mayo Clinic guys! All you folks at Johns Hopkins! And the team down at the Salk Institute: We're a little tired of waiting for you to cure the common cold. Seriously, you knock out polio but you can't fix the sniffles? What's that about?

Well, to give you folks a hand, we've decided to bring in a second opinion from a leading scientist in the field of immunology and otolaryngology: my mom. With more than 40 years of experience caring for obstinate children who refused to wear hats while waiting for the school bus, she has developed her own magical elixir to win the war on the common cold: soup.

BOGUS LABEL ALERT! *"1 cup." Most soups list 1 cup as a serving (some even less), but you know and I know (and they know) that most of us don't eat half a container of soup; we pour the whole thing in a bowl, nuke it, and off we go. So figure that whatever you're reading on the label is actually twice as good—or twice as bad.*

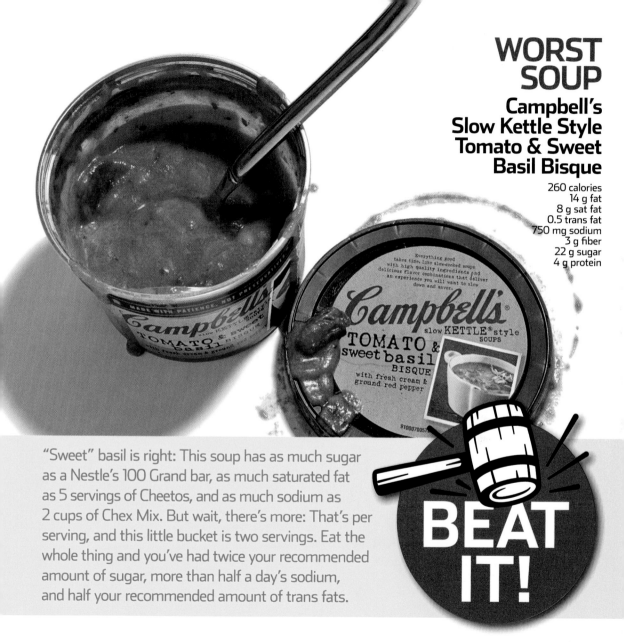

WORST SOUP

Campbell's Slow Kettle Style Tomato & Sweet Basil Bisque

260 calories
14 g fat
8 g sat fat
0.5 trans fat
750 mg sodium
3 g fiber
22 g sugar
4 g protein

"Sweet" basil is right: This soup has as much sugar as a Nestle's 100 Grand bar, as much saturated fat as 5 servings of Cheetos, and as much sodium as 2 cups of Chex Mix. But wait, there's more: That's per serving, and this little bucket is two servings. Eat the whole thing and you've had twice your recommended amount of sugar, more than half a day's sodium, and half your recommended amount of trans fats.

BEAT IT!

And research, for once, backs her up. (Which is not what happened when she tried to teach me about the birds and the bees. You can't go blind that way, Mom!) Mom's homemade chicken soup has even been shown to interact with white blood cells and improve immune function. But if you don't have time to make soup at home, make sure you have the right store-bought brands on hand.

THE SOUP RULES

DON'T GET TOO SALTY. The FDA recommends we consume no more than 2,400 mg of sodium per day, but some soups can contain up to 1,800 mg per cup—and a bowl of it can blow your daily allowance. Try to keep your sodium under 500 mg per serving.

ROUGHAGE YOURSELF UP. The high water content in soup helps keep you full, but so does the high fiber content; look for at least 2 g fiber.

KNOW BEANS. Beans are just about the perfect weight-loss food, packed with protein, fiber, and antioxidants. But it's not like you can just keep a jar of black-eyed peas on your desk. Soups are one of the best places to find them.

ROOT FOR THE YANKEES. Creamy soups are higher in calories and fat. Always pick the Manhattan clam chowder over the New England.

THE SOUP ADVANTAGE

Lose Weight

America's favorite flavors, to no surprise, are tomato and chicken noodle—and, in the right serving size, both can be a great addition to a meal. According to a Penn State study, consuming low-calorie soup (broth based, not creamy) as a first course can cut total calorie intake at a meal by 20 percent.

Boost Immunity

A study conducted by the Nebraska Medical Center used blood samples from volunteers and found that chicken soup helps reduce upper respiratory cold symptoms.

BEST SOUP

Amy's Organic Light in Sodium Lentil Vegetable

160 calories
4 g fat
0.5 g sat fat
340 mg sodium
8 g fiber
5 g sugar
7g protein

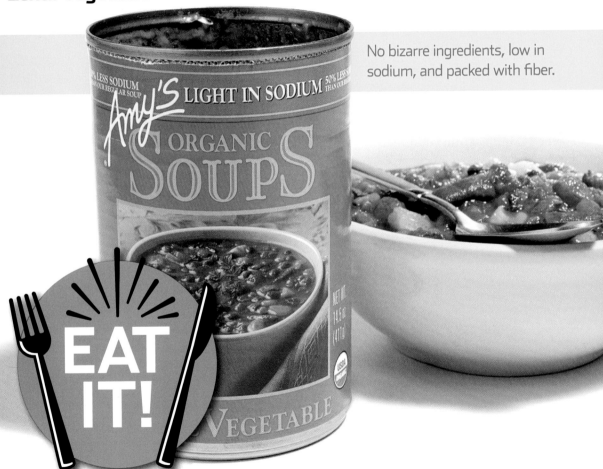

No bizarre ingredients, low in sodium, and packed with fiber.

EAT IT!

AMY'S ORGANIC
Light in Sodium Butternut Squash Soup

- 100 calories
- 2 g fat
- 0 g sat fat
- 290 mg sodium
- 2 g fiber
- 4 g sugar
- 2 g protein

PACIFIC ORGANIC
Vegetable Lentil & Roasted Red Pepper Reduced Sodium

- 150 calories
- 0.5 g fat
- 0 g sat fat
- 490 mg sodium
- 7 g fiber
- 5 g sugar
- 8 g protein

TABATCHNICK
Black Bean Soup

- 220 calories
- 2.5 g fat
- 0 g sat fat
- 400 mg sodium
- 9 g fiber
- 2 g sugar
- 13 g protein

Whole foods, no additives, low sugar!

PROGRESSO
Light Savory Vegetable Barley

- 60 calories
- 0 fat
- 0 sat fat
- 480 mg sodium
- 4 g fiber
- 2 g sugar
- 2 g protein

More ingredients than we'd like to see, but at least most of them are pronounceable

CAMPBELL'S
Homestyle Chicken Noodle Soup

- 70 calories
- 2 g fat
- 0.5 g sat fat
- 940 mg of sodium
- 1 g fiber
- 1 g sugar
- 3 g protein

Look out! A serving size is only ½ cup, so even if you enjoy a single cup of soup, you're at 80 percent of your daily sodium intake.

AMY'S
Cream of Mushroom

- 150 calories
- 9 g fat
- 2 g sat fat
- 590 mg sodium
- 2 g fiber
- 3 g sugar
- 3 g protein
- *In ¾ cup*

More sugar than fiber, and serving size is less than a cup

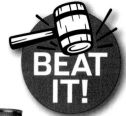

PROGRESSO
High Fiber Creamy Tomato Basil

- 130 calories
- 3.5 g fat
- 1 g sat fat
- 690 mg sodium
- 7 g fiber
- 13 g sugar
- 2 g protein

Twice as much sugar as fiber

HEALTHY CHOICE
Hearty Chicken Soup

- 130 calories
- 2 g fat
- 0.5 g sat fat
- 480 mg sodium
- 3 g fiber
- 2 g sugar
- 8 g protein

Looks like a healthy profile but . . . why is there turkey fat in my chicken soup? Not to mention soy protein, potassium chloride, thiamine mononitrate, ferrous sulfate, disodium insinuate, calcium chloride . . . you get the idea.

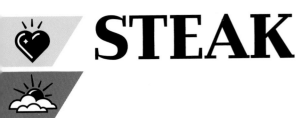

STEAK

It's the turf in your surf-and-turf, the meat in your meat-and-potatoes. It's the go-to meal for celebrating a big score, the ultimate affordable American luxury, the red-blood-and-muscle-building dinnertime backbone of red-blooded Americans.

It's also the bane of vegans, environmentalists, and cardiologists around the world, who swear that if we'd just stopped eating steak, we'd end animal cruelty, stop global warming, prevent mad-cow disease, and maybe have fewer heart attacks along the way. How did such a perfect food, so richly marbled and delicious, become so politically fraught? Don't worry, I'm here to break the political gridlock—maybe with a nice merlot . . .

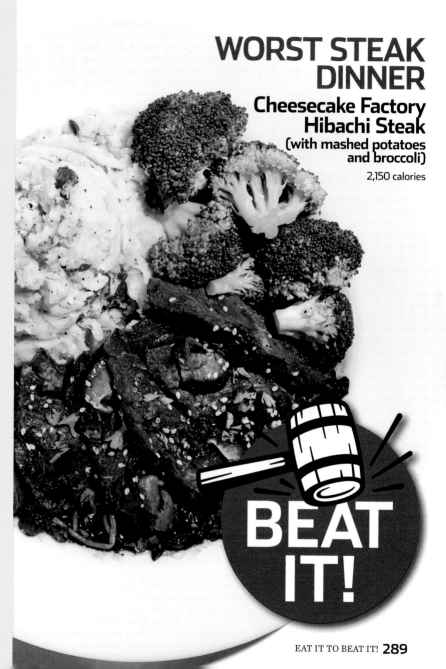

Better just have a glass of water with this meal because you can't afford any more calories. Consisting of Certified Angus hanger steak with shiitake mushrooms, onions, bean sprouts, wasabi mashed potatoes, and broccoli, it sounds like a healthy balance of meat, carbs, and vegetables . . . but don't be fooled. This meal will put you over your calorie limit for the entire day.

WORST STEAK DINNER

Cheesecake Factory Hibachi Steak

(with mashed potatoes and broccoli)

2,150 calories

BEAT IT!

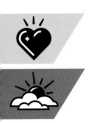
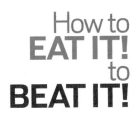

How to EAT IT! to BEAT IT!

Before you start a Political Action Committee to battle the pro- or anti-beef forces, here are a few things to consider.

- In moderation, steak is good for you and provides a great source of vitamins and minerals, as well as protein.
- Eating too much is bad for you, and can lead to diabetes, heart disease, and other nasty issues.
- Eating too much or too little can lead to depression.
- Beef is kinda bad for the environment, that's true. About 8 percent of greenhouse gasses come from beef farming. The other 92 percent come from transportation, electricity, and other commercial and residential activity. So if climate change is your game, you'll make more of a positive impact if you bike to the butcher, then eat your steak by candlelight.
- There are some trace amounts of antibiotics and synthetic hormones in most beef. Grass-fed, organic beef is healthier for you because it's free of these substances and higher in healthy omega-3 fatty acids, but it is also more expensive.

THE STEAK RULES

EAT STEAK AT HOME PLATE. A steak dinner ought to be around 500 calories, and it's not hard to cook yourself. But a steak dinner at a sit-down chain restaurant is almost always going to cost you at least 1,000 calories (and that's before your beverage, bread basket, and desert are factored in). That's because restaurants often coat the steaks with butter to make them glisten like Katy Perry's lip gloss.

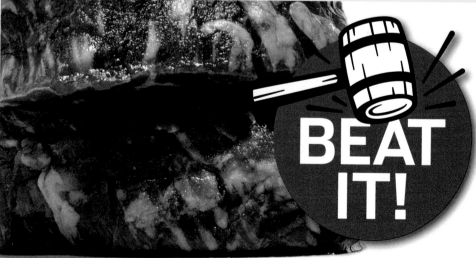

WORST SUPERMARKET STEAK

Sam's Club Kobe Beef of Texas Filet
(8 oz./6 pk.)

Kobe beef comes only from a certain breed of cow, called the Wagyu, which is raised only in certain parts of Japan. So what is Sam's Club charging you $252.88 for? Imitation Kobe. While the Texans might be trying to replicate some of the pampering the Japanese perform on their Wagyu cows, American Kobe-Style beef often comes from American Angus cows that have been crossbred with American-raised Wagyu cows.

BEAT IT!

AVOID THE RADURA. Most of the meat at your local grocery store has probably been blasted with a bit of ionizing radiation to reduce microbial content and extend shelf life (of course, only as much radiation as the USDA deems safe, which is about 4.5 kilograys). But it has to be labeled. Since no food marketer wants the word "radiation" anywhere near their product, they'll often just use the Radura flower label (at left). Studies have found that irradiating meat can reduce some vitamin levels by as much as 50 percent.

GIVE IT THE SNIFF TEST. Supermarket beef is usually treated with carbon monoxide to keep its red color, which means it can go bad and still look good. The only way to tell if beef has gone bad is to smell it. Rancid meat smells vaguely of cottage cheese.

 GO ASK ANGUS. While finding grass-fed, local, pasture-raised beef might be the best option, if you can find the Certified Black Angus Natural label (at left), you're getting the best choice and prime grades of beef, plus these cows have never been given antibiotics or added hormones.

Quick Chart

Scary things that weigh 100 pounds

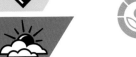

Gray wolf

HAL-3 hellfire missile

12 gallons of gasoline

Baby hippopotamus

American's annual red-meat intake

107 lbs, actually

THE STEAK ADVANTAGE

Lower Cholesterol

A recent study in the *American Journal of Clinical Nutrition* found that including 4 ounces of lean beef (select-grade top round, chuck shoulder pot roast, and 95 percent lean ground beef) per day can decrease total cholesterol by 4 percent and decrease LDL cholesterol by 5 percent.

Improve Mood

An Australian study found that women who cut red meat from their diet are more likely to suffer from anxiety and depression. The study also found that getting more than the recommended 3 ounces of red meat per day increased their risk for depression.

CANDY COWS

Grain-fed beef. Sounds wholesome, right? Feedlot cows are fed a mixture of corn and soy, but as corn prices have increased, so have reports of farmers supplementing cows' diets with ice cream sprinkles, marshmallows, and even gummy worms. But don't worry: Since these candies are made primarily of corn sweeteners and soybean oils, these can still be called "grain-fed beef." Now go and finish up your gummy worms, or there will be no dessert for you!

BEST STEAK DINNER

Longhorn Steakhouse
Flo's Filet 7 oz
(with side of green beans)

460 calories
30 g fat
602 mg sodium
7 g carbs
41 g protein

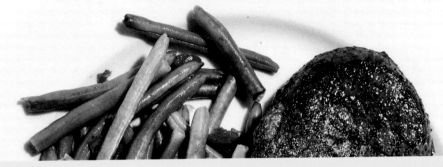

There might be one or two steak meals out there with fewer calories, but they all have about a thousand more mgs of sodium, or they are a subpar cut of beef. Longhorn Steakhouse does the best job of delivering a quality cut with a reasonable nutritional profile.

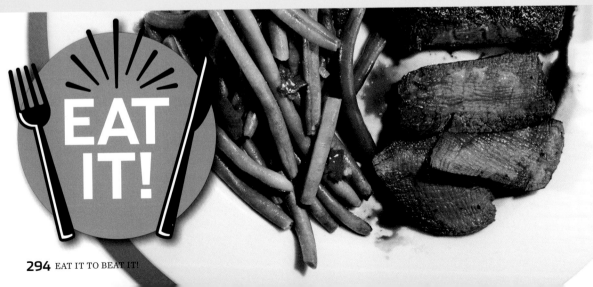

EAT IT!

TGI FRIDAY'S

Sirloin
6 oz, (with mashed potatoes and broccoli)

630 calories
34.5 g fat
2,360 mg sodium
8 g fiber
44 g protein

UNO CHICAGO GRILL

Top Sirloin
8 oz

410 calories
14 g fat
1,320 mg sodium
0 g fiber
66 g protein

CHILI'S

Classic Sirloin
6 oz (with mashed potatoes and steamed broccoli)

890 calories
50 g fat
2,270 mg sodium
9 g fiber
52 g protein

OUTBACK STEAKHOUSE

Outback Special Sirloin
6 oz (with house salad and garlic mashed potatoes)

940 calories
61 g fat
1,887 mg sodium
9 g fiber
13 g sugar
50 g protein

APPLEBEE'S

House Sirloin
9 oz (served with baked potato and seasonal vegetables)

1,000 calories
13 g fat
1,070 mg sodium
1 g fiber
44 g protein

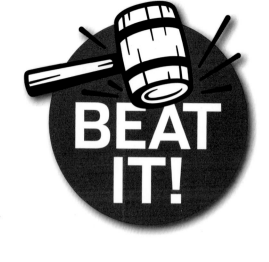

OUTBACK STEAKHOUSE

Porterhouse Steak
(with fries and house salad with ranch dressing)

1,815 calories
128 g fat
2,724 mg sodium
7 g fiber
108 g protein

CHEESECAKE FACTORY

Crispy Spicy Beef
1,530 calories
Further information n/a

HARD ROCK CAFE

New York Strip Steak
1,502 calories
Further information n/a

ROMANO'S MACARONI GRILL

Chianti BBQ Steak
1,920 calories
121 g fat
3,130 mg sodium
9 g fiber
120 g protein

LONGHORN

Porterhouse
1,200 calories
85 g fat
4 g trans fat
2,180 mg sodium

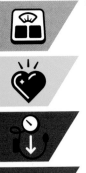

VEGETARIAN ENTREES & MEAT SUBSTITUTES

You'd think that when choosing vegetarian meat substitutes, finding healthy options would be a cinch. After all, you're swapping the butchered flesh of a poor, defenseless animal for the natural gifts directly from Mother Earth. Slap on the Birkenstocks, fire up the Subaru, and let's go shopping!

But it's not that simple. Most vegetarian foods are made for people who hate being vegetarian—self-loathing herbivores who want nothing more than to gnaw meat from bone but choose not to for medical, ethical, environmental, or religious reasons, or because they accidentally saw that *Food, Inc.* movie and can't look at a hot dog without a straight-up Pavlovian panic attack.

So while eating a vegetarian diet is healthy, eating a lot of "vegetarian" foods—as opposed to actual vegetables—isn't always the best option. Most meat substitutes are more like diskettes of water mixed with chemicals—sort of the vegetarian version of the BP oil spill.

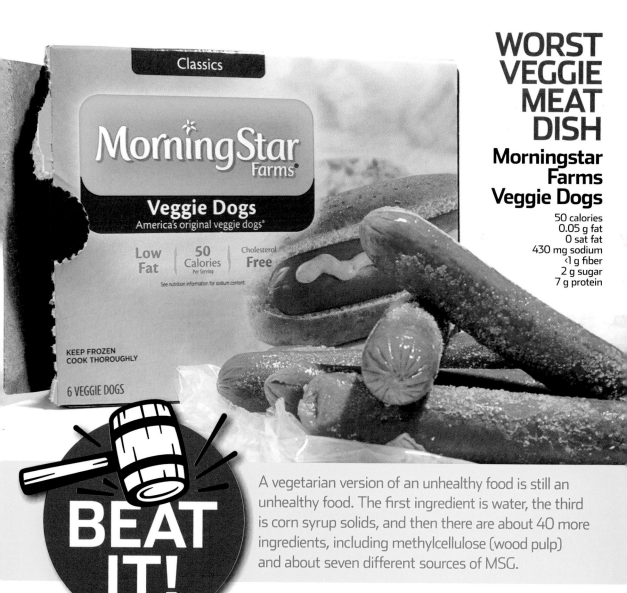

Classics

MorningStar Farms®

Veggie Dogs
America's original veggie dogs®

Low Fat | 50 Calories Per Serving | Cholesterol Free

See nutrition information for sodium content.

KEEP FROZEN
COOK THOROUGHLY

6 VEGGIE DOGS

WORST VEGGIE MEAT DISH

Morningstar Farms Veggie Dogs

50 calories
0.05 g fat
0 sat fat
430 mg sodium
<1 g fiber
2 g sugar
7 g protein

BEAT IT!

A vegetarian version of an unhealthy food is still an unhealthy food. The first ingredient is water, the third is corn syrup solids, and then there are about 40 more ingredients, including methylcellulose (wood pulp) and about seven different sources of MSG.

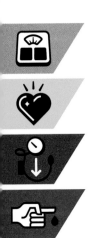

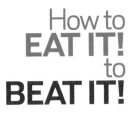

How to **EAT IT!** to **BEAT IT!**

In July of 2013, the *JAMA Internal Medicine* published a study that found vegetarians live longer than meat-eaters. The researchers tracked about 73,000 members of the Seventh Day Adventist church, a religious sect that advocates vegetarian eating, although not all members follow that teaching. Researchers found out what type of diet each person ate, then followed up with participants periodically over six years, noting how many people died and how they died. Vegetarians in the study experienced 12 percent fewer deaths over the period.

THE VEGGIE BURGER RULES

DON'T GET WATERED DOWN. You'll see that many of these products list "water" as the first ingredient, which is how they keep their calorie counts down. But water isn't what you want between the hamburger rolls.

DON'T BAT 400. Meat substitutes can be high in sodium. Look to stay under 400 mg of sodium per serving.

GO NAKED. Breading on real meat is a bad idea, and the same holds true for meat substitutes. It's where the hidden trans fats live.

PLAY WITH PROTEINS. Soy remains a bit controversial because the naturally occurring compounds in the bean are "estrogenic," meaning they mimic the effects of estrogen. Fine in small quantities, not fine if it's the basis of every meal. So while tofu and tempeh are healthy options, look for other sources of protein, including beans and mushrooms.

THE VEGETARIAN ADVANTAGE

Lower Cholesterol

A Korean study published in the journal *Nutrition Research and Practice* in 2012 found that vegetarian eaters had significantly lower levels of total cholesterol and LDL "bad" cholesterol. Another study, published in the *American Journal of Clinical Nutrition* in March of 2013, found that vegetarians had a 32 percent lower risk for hospitalization or death from heart disease.

Lower Blood Pressure

In a 2012 study of Seventh Day Adventists published in the journal *Public Health Nutrition*, researchers concluded that vegetarians, and especially vegans, have lower blood pressure and less hypertension than omnivores.

Beat Diabetes

A 2013 study published in the journal *Nutrition, Metabolism and Cardiovascular Diseases* found a "substantial and independent" reduction in risk for diabetes in people who ate a vegetarian diet.

Lose Weight

Many studies have found a relationship between lower body weight and a vegetarian diet. A 2011 study published in the *Journal of the Academy of Nutrition and Dietetics* took up this question and concluded that vegetarian diets "are nutrient dense, consistent with dietary guidelines, and could be recommended for weight management."

BEST VEGGIE BURGER

Quorn Turk'y Burger

90 calories
4 g fat
0.5 g sat fat
200 mg sodium
2 g fiber
0 g sugar
10 g protein

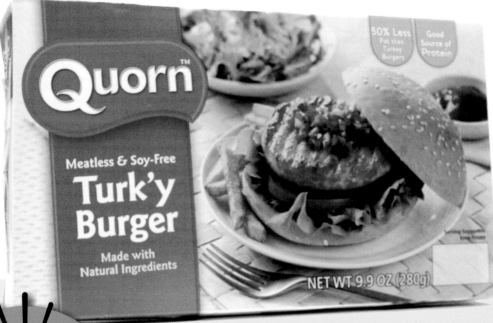

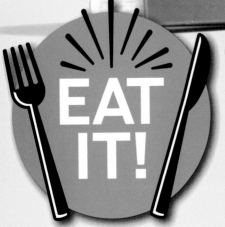

Quorn is made primarily from mycoprotein, a fungus-based protein that's grown in vats of glucose. But if you can get beyond the science-fiction aspect of Quorn, you'll discover a product that's free of estrogen-mimicking soy and many of the additives that other vegetarian dishes need to keep them fresh. The best of the Quorn line is the Turk'y Burger, which contains little more than the mycoprotein, some egg white, wheat flour, and canola oil.

MORNINGSTAR FARMS
Original Grillers

130 calories
6 g fat
1 g sat fat
260 mg sodium
2 g fiber
1 g sugar
15 g protein

Higher in protein and lower in sodium than many brands

QUORN
Meatballs

90 calories
1.5 g fat
0.5 g sat fat
390 mg sodium
1 g fiber
1 g sugar
13 g protein

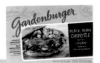

GARDENBURGER
Black Bean Chipotle Veggie Burger

90 calories
3 g fat
0 g sat fat
390 mg sodium
4 g fiber
3 g sugar
5 g protein

A longer ingredient list than you'd normally want to see, but its protein comes primarily from beans and rice.

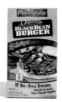

MORNINGSTAR FARMS
Chipotle Black Bean Burger

190 calories
7 g fat
1 g sat fat
540 mg sodium
8 g fiber
2 g sugar
17 g protein

Plenty of fiber and protein, but more sodium than a Taco Bell Fiery Doritos Locos Taco.

BOCA
Soy Protein Breakfast Sausage Links

70 calories
3 g fat
1 g sat fat
330 mg sodium
2 g fiber
2 g sugar
8 g protein

Low in calories, but low in everything else except additives

Spicy Chik'n Patties

160 calories
6 g fat
1 g sat fat
430 mg sodium
2 g fiber
1 g sugar
11 g protein

Water is the first ingredient.

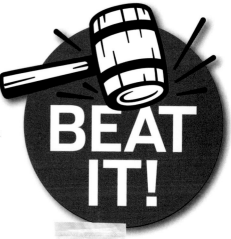

BEAT IT!

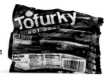

LIGHTLIFE BACKYARD
Grill'n Burgers

190 calories
9 g fat
0.5 g sat fat
350 mg sodium
1 g fiber
1 g sugar
20 g protein

Good stats, but again, it's in part because the first ingredient is water.

TOFURKY
Hot Dogs

100 calories
4.5 g fat
0 g sat fat
330 mg sodium
1 g fiber
2 g sugar
10 g protein

Two of the first three ingredients are water and canola oil.

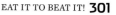

YOGURT

Long ago, before the invention of the wheel, or the wheel of cheese, a Neolithic tribe figured out how to milk their cows. Because they kept the milk in containers made from animal stomachs, the milk was exposed to natural enzymes, which curdled the milk and turned it into an early type of yogurt.

At least that's what anthropologists believe—the story is a little fuzzy, much like yogurt when it's left open in the fridge for too long. And thanks to food-manufacturer mischief, the facts surrounding this once-simple food are only getting fuzzier.

Stonyfield Farm Organic Vanilla Over Chocolate

170 calories
0 g fat
100 mg sodium
34 g sugar
7 g protein

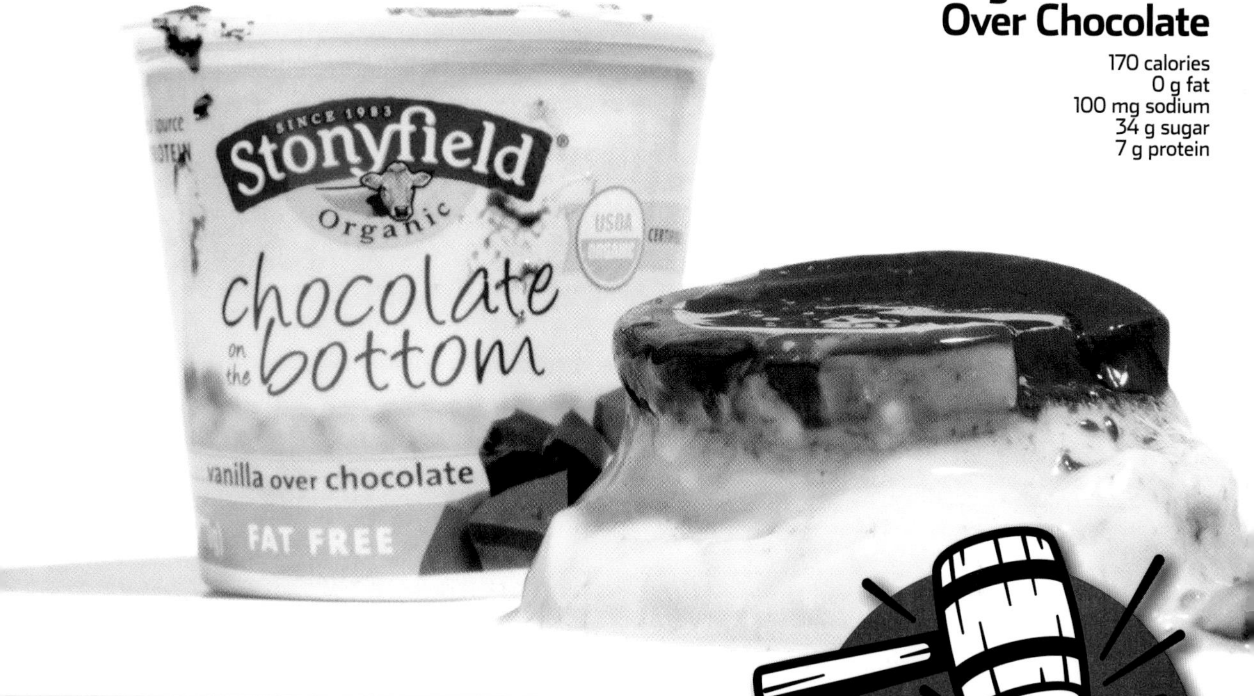

It's really Vanilla Over Chocolate Over Sugar.
It may be fat-free and organic, but it has as much sugar
as 7 Chips Ahoy! Chewy chocolate chip cookies.

BEAT IT!

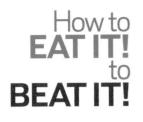

How to
EAT IT!
to
BEAT IT!

Over time, yogurt went from curdling in animal stomachs to being a 7.3-billion-dollar industry in the United States alone, one that's growing along with yoga studios, spinning classes, and the geriatric urgings of Jamie Lee Curtis's small intestine. But tread ye carefully in the aisle of the fermented milk products.

THE YOGURT RULES

BALANCE PROTEIN AND SUGAR. The best yogurts have a sugar-to-protein ratio of about 1:1. The worst? About 5:1.

DISPUTE THE FRUIT. "Fruit on the Bottom" often means "sugar on the top." Make sure that all sugars are accounted for in the ingredient list and none come from sugar or high fructose corn syrup. The healthiest yogurt is always a plain yogurt to which you add your own fruit.

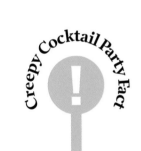

Creepy Cocktail Party Fact

There are
10 times
as many
bacteria cells
in your body as
there are
human cells.

TRY GREEK LIFE. Both regular and Greek yogurts are healthy options, but the Greek variety has an undeniable edge: In roughly the same amount of calories, Greek yogurt has double the protein and far less sugar.

BEAT THE HEAT. By law, manufacturers can call something yogurt only if there are these two strains of live, active cultures added: *Lactobacillus bulgaricus* and *Streptococcus thermophilus* (collectively, these good-for-you bacteria are known as acidophilus). However, some yogurts are heat-treated after fermentation, which can kill off the good-for-you bacteria required for production. If your yogurt is not heat-treated, the package may say "active yogurt cultures," "living yogurt cultures," or "contains active cultures."

THE YOGURT ADVANTAGE

Lose Weight

A 2012 study published in the *International Journal of Obesity* found that obese adults who ate three servings of fat-free yogurt each day as part of a reduced-calorie diet lost 22 percent more weight and 61 percent more body fat compared to those that didn't have yogurt.

Beat Diabetes

Plain yogurt has a glycemic index of just 14, which means it has little effect on blood sugar. A landmark review published in the journal *Diabetes Care* concluded that diets high in calcium from foods like yogurt, reduce the risk for type 2 diabetes by 33 percent.

Boost Immunity

Because yogurt is made with fermented milk, it contains "good" bacteria that may boost your immune system. A Taiwanese study found that yogurt containing two probiotics, *lactobacillus* and *bifidobacterium,* improved the success of drug therapy in 138 people with persistent ulcers.

BEST YOGURT

Siggi's Icelandic Style Skyr Strained Non-Fat Yogurt Vanilla

Siggi's isn't a Greek yogurt, but it's made in a similar way, which helps to up the protein value. Plain yogurts will have the least sugar, but among flavored options this may be the healthiest.

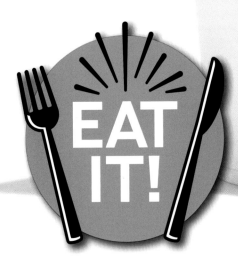

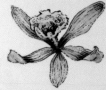

siggi's®

Icelandic style skyr | **0%** Milkfat | strained non-fat yogurt

VANILLA

9g Sugar | 14g Protein | 100 Calories

100 calories
0 g fat
60 mg sodium
9 g sugar
14 g protein

WALLABY
Organic Greek Lowfat with Blueberries
140 calories
2.5 g fat
85 mg sodium
15 g sugar
12 g protein

YOPLAIT
Greek 100 Calories
100 calories
0 g fat
45 mg sodium
9 g sugar
10 g protein

STONYFIELD
Organic Greek Blueberry
120 calories
0 g fat
70 mg sodium
15 g sugar
13 g protein

CHOBANI
Champions Tubes Jammin' Strawberry
70 calories
1 g fat
25 mg sodium
8 g sugar
5 g protein

DANNON
Light & Fit Greek
80 calories
0 g fat
45 mg sodium
8 g sugar
12 g protein

FAGE
Fruyo 0% Blueberry
140 calories
0 g fat
50 mg sodium
20 g sugar
14 g protein

DANNON
All Natural Vanilla
160 calories
2.5 g fat
105 mg sodium
25 g sugar
8 g protein

With three times as much sugar as protein, this is more like ice cream than yogurt.

Activia Vanilla
110 calories
2 g fat
60 mg sodium
17 g sugar
4 g protein

Sugar, fructose, and modified cornstarch all boost the carb content.

Light & Fit Carb & Sugar Control
45 calories
1.5 g fat
25 mg sodium
2 g sugar
5 g protein

The diet soda of yogurts, with sucralose, and a number of unpronounceables

YOPLAIT
Thick and Creamy Strawberry Banana
180 calories
2.5 g fat
110 mg sodium
28 g sugar
7 g protein

Four times as much sugar as protein

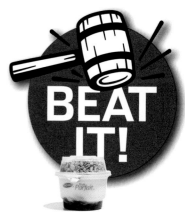

BEAT IT!

YOCRUNCH
Parfait Vanilla Nonfat Yogurt with Strawberries and Lowfat Granola
110 calories
0.5 g fat
55 mg sodium
16 g sugar
3 g protein

Fruit parfait? More like sugar with red 40

HORIZON
Organic Tuberz Surfin' Strawberry
60 calories
0.5 g fat
40 mg sodium
10 g sugar
2 g protein

Very little protein, thanks to sugar being the second ingredient and 9 more ingredients after that

COOK IT TO BEAT IT!

By now you're probably a little freaked out by the tricks restaurants and packaged-food marketers have been using to put our food on steroids.

I know I am. Today's meals, snacks, and desserts feel less like actual foods and more like chemical experiments out of a demented Tim Burton movie—and the guinea pigs are you and me.

We don't know for sure what all these concoctions are doing to our bodies, but we do know one thing: We're just

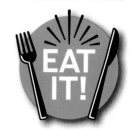

not as lean, fit, and healthy as we ought to be. Every commercial interruption of *America's Got Talent* seems to be for a prescription drug that helps us lower cholesterol, lose weight, fight migraines, beat allergies, overcome depression, or perform some other medical trick we didn't seem to need 20 years ago. (Side effects may include drowsiness, irritability, and growing a second head. . . .)

It's too bad, because the original medicine—the stuff that has been curing our troubles and fighting off our diseases since the time of the caveman—isn't found in your medicine chest. It's found in your refrigerator. Healthy, vitamin-and-mineral-packed whole foods are the most potent weapons we have against everyday ills. And the more control you have over the foods you eat—the more you can cook yourself and keep your food intake unadulterated by additional chemicals and bizarre ingredients—the more you know you're treating your body right. After all, if you had a cold, you wouldn't just wander into the drug store, buy whatever pills you came across, and randomly down a handful of them without reading the labels, would you? ("Why not?" says Keith Richards. . . .)

Instead, you'd carefully select the medicines that were best for your individual health concerns.

Well, that's what you should do with your meals. Instead of trusting manufacturers to pour an indiscriminate concoction of food (and food-like) substances into your body, you can take back control of your life and your well-being if you simply learn a hand-ful of go-to recipes that are just as delicious as anything you'll find in a chain restaurant—but that give your body the weapons it needs to stay lean, strong, and healthy.

Here, I've collected some of my favorite super-easy, super-healthy recipes. Each one will help bolster your overall health and well-being. Here's how you can . . .

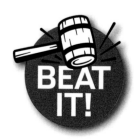

BANISH BRAIN FOG

BEAT IT!

Some anthropologists believe that simpleminded Neanderthals evolved into the super-sophisticated *Pawn Stars*–watching intellectuals we are today once they moved closer to the sea and began eating omega-3-rich seafood. This heart-and-brain-healthy food has been shown to improve cognitive function, while brightly colored foods provide micronutrients that protect the brain against premature aging. Researchers from the National Institutes of Health and the National Institute on Aging found that people with diets high in omega-3 fatty acids, and in vitamins C, D, E, and B, score higher on mental thinking tests than people with diets that are low in those nutrients. They also found that omega-3s protect against the brain shrinkage associated with Alzheimer's.

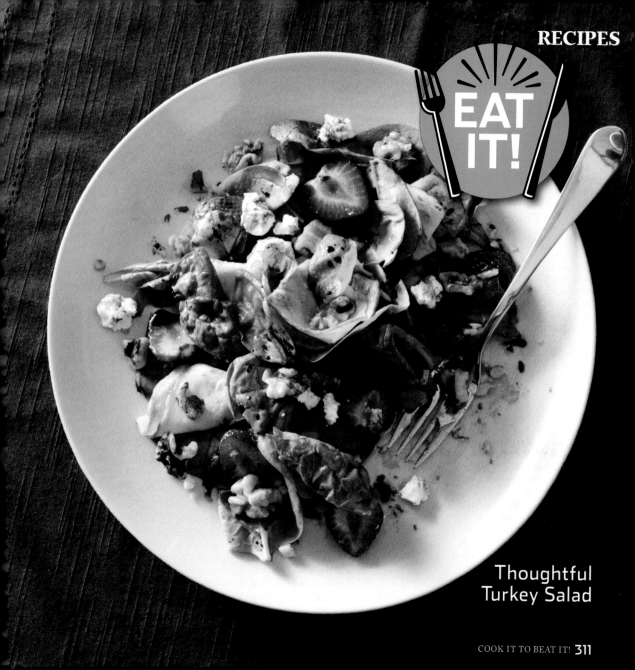

EAT IT!

Thoughtful
Turkey Salad

THE RED, WHITE, & BLUE BRAIN

The key to this brainy, patriotic breakfast is in its color. Blue, red, and purple fruits and vegetables contain anthocyanins, a form of antioxidant known to improve neuronal and cognitive function.

½ cup frozen blueberries

½ cup frozen strawberries

½ cup pomegranate juice

½ cup 2% Greek yogurt

▼

Combine all ingredients in a blender and puree until smooth and uniform.

MAKES 1 SERVING

210 calories / 3 g fat / 1.5 g sat fat / 50 mg sodium / 4 g fiber / 30 g sugar / 10 g protein

Thoughtful Turkey Salad

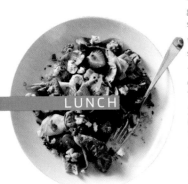

LUNCH

8 cups baby spinach

½ cup sliced strawberries

¼ cup fresh goat cheese or feta, crumbled

2 Tbsp walnuts (best when toasted)

2 ounces smoked turkey, torn into thin slices

1 Tbsp olive oil

½ Tbps balsamic vinegar

It's no mere coincidence that walnuts are shaped like little brains. With dense reserves of brain-boosting omega-3s, a cache of anti-inflammatory polyphenols, and the ability to dramatically increase levels of serotonin (a nutrient vital for sound sleep), walnuts may do as much for your noggin as any other food out there. They may be the star of this salad, but turkey, loaded with choline, and strawberries, an excellent source of flavonoids, will help keep you sharp, too. Most important, the combination of sweet, creamy, crunchy, smoky ingredients makes for a heroic midday meal.

▼

In a large mixing bowl, combine the spinach, strawberries, cheese, walnuts, and turkey. Drizzle with olive oil and vinegar and season to taste with salt and pepper.

MAKES 1 SERVING

520 calories
37 g fat
11 g sat fat
940 mg sodium
8 g fiber
6 g sugar
34 g protein

DINNER

SMOKY SALMON SYNAPSE SHARPENER

When it comes to sharpening memory and cognitive function, reams of research have shown that nothing gets the job done quite like omega-3s. And when it comes to omega-3s, nothing packs these vital fatty acids quite like wild salmon. This Mediterranean treatment pairs smoky spices with the cooling effect of Greek yogurt, which—with a drizzle of olive oil and a bit of garlic and herbs—makes a versatile sauce for grilled chicken, pork chops, or fish. Serve this over couscous studded with toasted pine nuts, golden raisins, and cilantro.

1 cup 2% Greek yogurt

1 Tbsp olive oil

1 clove garlic, finely minced

½ medium cucumber, peeled, seeded, and finely minced

Juice of half a lemon

Fresh chopped dill, parsley, or cilantro

Salt and black pepper to taste

4 4-oz filets wild salmon

½ tsp cumin

½ tsp paprika (preferably Spanish-style smoked paprika)

Preheat the oven to 475°F.

In a medium mixing bowl, combine the yogurt, oil, garlic, cucumber, lemon juice, and herbs, plus salt to taste. Set aside.

Season the salmon filets with cumin, paprika, and salt and pepper to taste. Place on a baking sheet and cook in the middle rack of the oven for 8 to 10 minutes, until the fish flakes with gentle pressure from your finger. Serve with the tzatziki.

MAKES 4 SERVINGS

130 calories
20 g fat
4.5 g sat fat
85 g sodium
0 g fiber
3 g sugar
28 g protein

BOOST IMMUNITY

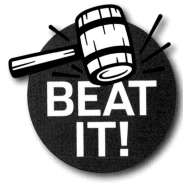

When it comes to granting yourself immunity, you need to become a man (or woman) of letters: vitamins A, B, C, D, E, and K, as well as minerals, play an enormous role in keeping your immune system strong. (No word on what happened to vitamins F and G, but we suspect Vladimir Putin had something to do with their disappearance.) And the best sources of these vitamins and minerals are nature's multivitamins, the cruciferous vegetables also known as arugula, bok choy, broccoli, Brussels sprouts, cabbage, cauliflower, collards, kale, kohlrabi, radishes, rutabaga, turnips, and watercress. A recent study in the journal *Cell* explained how these vegetables create a chemical signal that helps the immune cells in our guts and on our skin function properly. And more and more research is finding that the tiny microbes in our stomachs are the key to a healthy immune system.

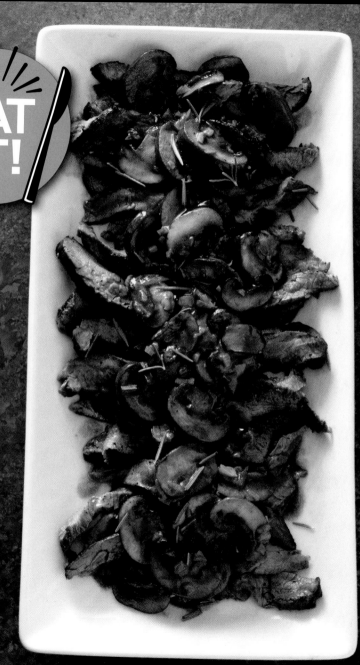

EAT
IT!

Trouble-
Skirting
Skirt Steak

THE C MONSTER

A morning megashot of vitamin C may provide the kind of daily fortification your body needs to function at the highest possible level. This simple smoothie hits the vitamin C trifecta: orange juice, pineapple chunks, and strawberries, three of the best sources of the vitamin on the planet. Feel like mixing it up from time to time? Kiwi, raspberries, and papaya are all excellent vitamin C sources as well. To add a cruciferous punch to this punch, throw in a few sprigs of watercress.

½ medium apple, roughly chopped	½ cup frozen pineapple
1 cup watercress (optional)	1 Tbsp fresh ginger (optional)
½ cup orange juice	½ cup Greek yogurt

Combine all ingredients in a blender and puree until smooth and uniform.

MAKES 1 SERVING

255 calories / 3 g fat / 1.5 g sat fat / 42 mg sodium / 4 g fiber / 32 g sugar / 11 g protein

All Kale Caesar

Romaine, the traditional star of this salad, is a perfectly healthy leaf, but kale contains one of the most powerful nutritional profiles you'll find in nature, including huge stores of vitamins A, C, and K, a mixture of B vitamins, and over 45 different disease-fighting flavonoids. Roasted red bell peppers add an extra hit of vitamin C (they pack nearly twice as much C as an orange), plus a ton of sweet, smoky flavor. Keep the core components the same, but feel free to improvise the supporting cast: Toasted almonds, grilled asparagus, and hard-boiled egg would all make worthy additions.

1 tsp Worcestershire sauce

1 tsp Dijon mustard

Juice of one lemon

1 Tbsp olive oil mayonnaise

1 clove garlic

1 filet anchovy (optional)

Black pepper to taste

¼ cup olive oil

1 bunch kale, shredded

2 cups cooked chicken (grilled chicken breast, leftover roast chicken, or a store-bought rotisserie chicken all work great)

½ cup jarred roasted red peppers

½ cup grated Parmesan cheese

Combine the Worcestershire, Dijon, lemon juice, mayonnaise, garlic, and anchovy (if using) in a food processor, along with a generous amount of black pepper. With the motor running, slowly drizzle in the olive oil until you have a smooth, emulsified dressing.

In a large salad bowl, combine the kale, chicken, red peppers, Parmesan, and dressing. Toss to evenly distribute the ingredients and let sit at least 15 minutes before serving (the extra time will help soften the kale).

MAKES 4 SERVINGS

380 calories
25 g fat
5 g sat fat
550 mg sodium
3 g fiber
1 g sugar
28 g protein

DINNER

Trouble-Skirting Skirt Steak

Mushrooms don't garner the type of nutritional fanfare that other fruits and vegetables do, but they're every bit the superfood. Beyond being a rich source of various B vitamins (vital for bolstering your immune system), mushrooms have also been shown in studies to reduce inflammation and protect against cardio-vascular disease. Mixed with red wine (which researchers from Harvard found can help protect against colds) and blanketed over a seared skirt steak (a rich source of zinc, and one of the best cuts of beef for your money), you can have a meal worthy of a steakhouse in under 20 minutes.

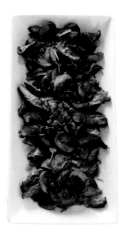

1 tsp olive oil

1 lb skirt, flank, or hanger steak

Salt and black pepper to taste

8 oz sliced cremini mushrooms

1 shallot, minced

1 clove garlic, minced

1 tsp all-purpose flour

½ cup chicken stock

½ cup red wine

1 Tbsp butter

Heat the olive oil in a large cast-iron or stainless steel pan over medium-high heat. Season the steak on both sides with salt and black pepper and place in the pan. Cook until nicely browned all over and firm but yielding to the touch, about 4 minutes per side. Remove to a cutting board to rest.

In the same pan (still set over medium-high heat), add the mushrooms, cook for a minute or two until softened, then add the shallot and garlic. Cook until the mushrooms are nicely browned, about 3 more minutes, then add the flour, stirring so it evenly coats the vegetables. Add the chicken stock and the red wine, whisking or stirring vigorously to prevent lumps from forming. Season with salt and black pepper to taste. At the last moment, swirl in the butter.

Slice the steak and divide among four warm plates. Divide the sauce among the four plates and serve.

MAKES 4 SERVINGS

CRUCIFY YOUR STEAK

To add a critical cruciferous punch to your steak-house feast, roughly chop up a pound of Brussels sprouts, lay them across a baking sheet, and lightly dress with olive oil, salt, and pepper. Bake at 400° F until lightly browned, about 25 minutes. Sprinkle a hand-ful of grated Parmesan over the sprouts during the last 5 min-utes of baking, if you'd like.

300 calories / 18 g fat / 7 g sat fat / 150 mg sodium / 0 g fiber / 2 g sugar / 26 g protein

COOK IT TO BEAT IT!

LOSE WEIGHT

BEAT IT!

All of the recipes in this chapter will help prevent weight gain. But if there's one thing that will have the biggest impact on your weight, it's this: Cut down on refined carbohydrates, such as white bread, sugar, and pastries. The three recipes here have one thing in common: They offer big, bold, satisfying flavor without relying on sweeteners or doughy carbs. Refined carbs are as addictive as drugs, which is why you can't stop eating them. The quick spike and crash in blood sugar that they cause activates the reward and addiction centers in your brain, causing you to crave and indulge. Plus, Harvard researchers found that reducing the amount of refined carb calories helps maintain weight loss better than reducing fat calories. In other words, not all calories are created equal, and refined carb calories are the worst for weight loss.

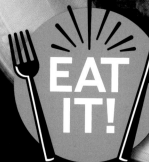

Green Eggs
& Ham

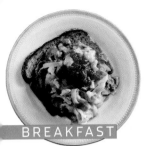

Green Eggs & Ham

1 tsp olive oil

2 large eggs

Salt to taste

2 Tbsp grated cheddar

2 thin slices deli ham, torn into strips

1 slice whole-wheat bread, toasted

1 Tbsp prepared guacamole (like Wholly Guacamole)

2 Tbsp bottled salsa

A study from Saint Louis University found that overweight people who consumed eggs in the morning felt greater satiety and consumed nearly 200 fewer calories at lunch than those who consumed bagels. This open-face sandwich might seem like a decadent start to your day, but it's exactly what your body needs.

▼

Heat the oil in a small nonstick pan over medium heat. Crack the eggs in a bowl, season with a few pinches of salt, and lightly whisk. Add the eggs to the pan, using a wooden spoon to stir the eggs and scrape the bottom of the pan, creating small, moist curds with the eggs. Add the cheddar and the ham, continuing to stir and scrape. When the eggs are just set, remove from the heat.

Slather the bread with the guacamole then add the scrambled eggs. Top with the salsa and eat.

MAKES 1 SERVING

430 calories
26 g fat
9 g sat fat
1,170 mg sodium
4 g fiber
3 g sugar
30 g protein

KEEN-WHAAA? SALAD

The Incas had it figured out over 500 years before the nutritionists: quinoa is one of the world's great superfoods. It has all the components of a weight-loss weapon: healthy fats, fiber, and nearly twice the protein of other grains.

Salt and black pepper to taste

1 cup dried quinoa

1 bunch asparagus, woody ends removed

1 Tbsp olive oil, plus more for drizzling

2 cups cooked chicken (grilled chicken breast,

leftover roast chicken, or a store-bough rotisserie chicken all work great)

¼ cup chopped sundried tomatoes

½ cup crumbled feta cheese

¼ cup store-bought pesto

1 Tbsp balsamic or red wine vinegar

▼

Preheat the oven to 450°F.

Bring a pot of water to boil, season with salt, and cook the quinoa until just al dente, about 20 minutes. Drain in a colander.

While the quinoa cooks, drizzle the asparagus with olive oil and season with salt and black pepper. Place in the oven and cook until gently browned and softened, about 10 to 12 minutes, depending on the thickness of the asparagus. Chop into bite-size pieces.

In a large mixing bowl, combine the quinoa with the chicken, asparagus, sundried tomatoes, and feta. Mix together the pesto, olive oil, and vinegar, then add it to the bowl of quinoa. Toss to combine.

MAKES 4 SERVINGS Keeps in the refrigerator for up to 5 days.

470 calories / 23 g fat / 7 g sat fat / 390 mg sodium / 4 g fiber / 5 g sugar / 34 g protein

Two to Tango Mango Tacos

DINNER

Blackening is the type of simple technique every cook should have in his or her arsenal—fast, easy, and one of the healthiest ways to infuse your food with big flavor. (All those spices? Zero-calorie vessels for antioxidants.) Here, the spicy shrimp (i.e. pure protein) team up with an A-list of nutritional superstars: avocado, mango, and black beans. Given how much flavor ends up cradled into those warm corn tortillas, you'd never guess it's exactly the kind of meal that will keep your body burning calories all night long.

1 ripe avocado, pitted and diced

1 mango, peeled and diced

½ medium red onion, diced

1 handful fresh cilantro, chopped

½ jalapeño, minced (optional)

Juice of one lime

Salt to taste

½ Tbsp olive or canola oil

1 lb medium shrimp, peeled and deveined

½ Tbsp blackening seasoning

8 corn tortillas, heated

1 cup canned black beans, heated

In a medium mixing bowl, combine the avocado, mango, onion, cilantro, and jalapeño, if using. Toss with the lime juice and season with salt to taste.

Heat the oil in a large grill pan, cast-iron skillet, or stainless steel pan over high heat. Coat the shrimp all over with the blackening seasoning. Add to the pan, cooking until firm to the touch and gently blackened on both sides, about 3 minutes total.

Place two warmed tortillas (you can use the same pan used to cook the shrimp to lightly toast them) on each of four plates. Top each with a spoonful of beans, a few shrimp, and a generous scoop of the mango-avocado salsa. Serve with more lime or hot sauce, if you like.

MAKES 4 SERVINGS

390 calories
12 g fat
2 g sat fat
940 mg sodium
12 g fiber
13 g sugar
24 g protein

LOWER CHOLESTEROL

If you want to lower your cholesterol naturally, remember the two Fs: fiber and healthy fats. Fiber keeps you fuller longer (cutting down on your tendency to snack on unhealthy foods) while ushering cholesterol out of your body. And the right kind of fats—monounsaturated fats from avocado, peanuts, olives, and the like—will change your cholesterol profile the way a newly single teenager changes her Facebook status. A recent study found that adding monounsaturated fats (MUFA) to your diet can increase good cholesterol (HDL) by 12.5 percent and lower LDL levels by 35 percent. And a Mediterranean-style diet, which is high in fruits, vegetables, and whole grains, low in red meat, and includes olive oil and moderate wine drinking, can lower your LDL cholesterol levels by 9 percent.

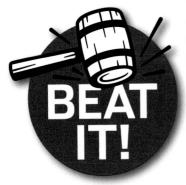

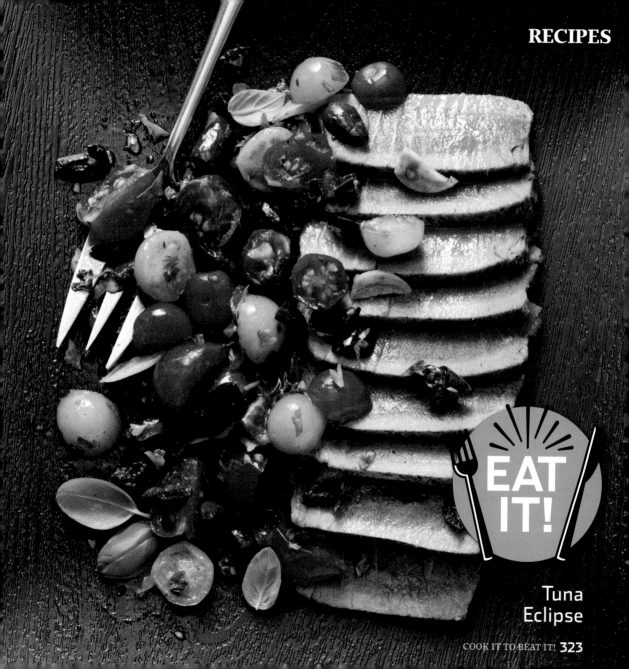

EAT
IT!

Tuna
Eclipse

Thin Elvis Oatmeal

Oats contain something called beta glucans, a form of soluble fiber that acts like your body's LDL bouncer, grabbing bad cholesterol trying to sneak into your system and kicking it to the curb. Stir in a generous spoonful of peanut butter (replete with heart-healthy fats) and sliced banana for natural sweetness and you have a powerful antidote to elevated cholesterol.

1 cup water

½ cup quick-cooking oats

1 Tbsp peanut butter

1 banana, sliced

Agave syrup or honey for sweetening (optional)

350 calories
11 g fat
2 g sat fat
90 mg sodium
8 g fiber
16 g sugar
10 g protein

▼

Bring the water to a boil. Stir in the oats and cook until soft, about 3 minutes. Just before the oats are finished, stir in the peanut butter, banana, and any additional sweetener you might like.

MAKES 1 SERVING

THE ALPHA OMEGA SANDWICH

A seminal review of studies published by the *American Journal of Clinical Nutrition* found that consuming omega-3 fatty acids could lower triglycerides by up to 30 percent. Cue smoked salmon, a potent source of omega-3s, and a natural partner with another source of healthy fat, fresh avocado. Throw in a bit of punchy wasabi-laced cream cheese and you have the kind of sandwich that works as well for breakfast as it does for lunch.

1 Tbsp whipped cream cheese

1 tsp prepared wasabi

2 slices sprouted-grain bread, lightly toasted

½ avocado, peeled, pitted, and sliced

2 thick slices tomato

2 oz smoked salmon

Sprouts

Combine the cream cheese and the wasabi in a mixing bowl and stir until evenly blended. Slather the mixture on one of the pieces of bread, then top with avocado, tomatoes, salmon, sprouts, and the remaining slice of bread.

MAKES 1 SERVING

430 calories / 24 g fat / 5 g sat fat / 780 mg sodium / 12 g fiber / 8 g sugar / 22 g protein

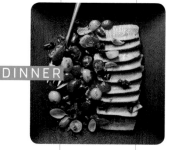

DINNER

Tuna Eclipse

The best way to combat bad cholesterol? Overwhelm it with the good stuff. Tuna, olive oil, and olives all contain the type of healthy fats that boost HDL levels, keeping those nasty LDL levels in check. This quick tomato sauce is normally served over spaghetti, but it's mixture of sweet and spicy flavors works even better over meaty slices of seared tuna.

▼

1 Tbsp olive oil

1 pint cherry tomatoes, halved

2 cloves garlic, sliced thin

Pinch red pepper flakes

½ cup roughly chopped kalamata olives

¼ cup dry red wine

10 leaves fresh basil, chopped

Salt and black pepper to taste

1 lb fresh tuna, like yellowfin or albacore

200 calories
6 g fat
1 g sat fat
180 mg sodium
1 g fiber
2 g sugar
29 g protein

Heat half the olive oil in a medium saucepan over medium heat. Add the tomatoes, garlic, and pepper flakes and cook until the tomatoes are softened and the garlic is lightly browned, about 5 minutes. Add the olives and red wine and cook until most of the wine has evaporated, another 3 minutes or so. Stir in the basil and season with salt and black pepper.

Heat the remaining oil in a grill pan, cast-iron skillet, or stainless steel saute pan over medium-high heat. Season the tuna on both sides with salt and pepper and place in the pan. Cook until nicely browned on the outside but still rare in the center, about 2 minutes per side.

Slice the tuna into ¼-inch slices. Divide among four plates and top with the puttanesca sauce.

MAKES 4 SERVINGS

LOWER BLOOD PRESSURE

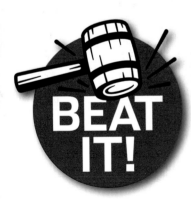

It's a myth that high blood pressure comes from too much sodium in your diet. Like all myths it has a bit of truth but it's more complicated than that. What really makes a difference is the ratio of sodium to other minerals—specifically potassium. Most Americans consume twice as much sodium as potassium, while doctors recommend consuming at least five times as much potassium as sodium. The problem: They don't sprinkle potassium on French fries. So you need not only to watch the salt but also to bump up your intake of potassium and other essential, good-for-you minerals. The American Heart Association estimates that increasing potassium intake would decrease the incidence of hypertension in Americans by 17 percent and would increase life expectancy by 5.1 years.

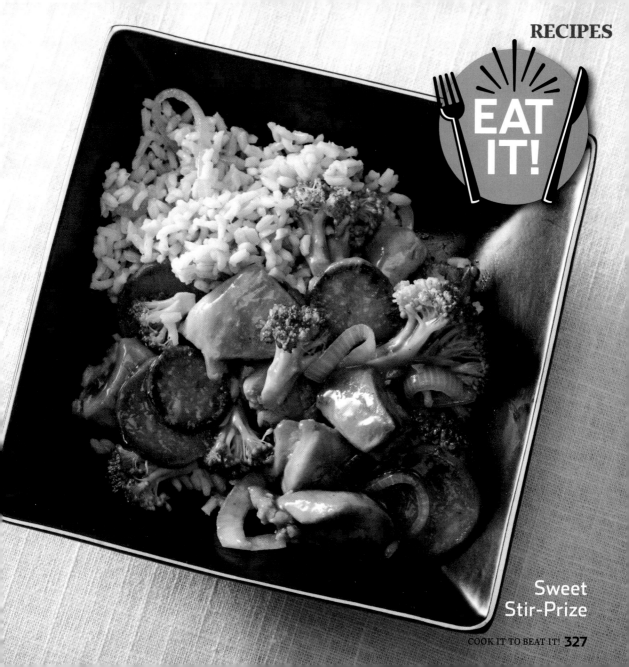

EAT IT!

Sweet
Stir-Prize

MR. CHILL'S BANANA-MANGO SMOOTHIE

There is no stress this morning: The 15-year Farmington Heart Study found that people who consume at least 2 percent of their daily calories from yogurt are 31 percent less likely to develop high blood pressure. Just another reason to make yogurt (especially Greek-style yogurt, which packs twice the amount of protein as the watery American stuff) the base of every smoothie you ever blend up. Throw in banana for a blast of potassium, some cubes of frozen mango for sweetness, and a bit of OJ for taste and texture and you have a drink to take the pressure off.

320 calories
3.5 g fat
2 g sat fat
40 mg sodium
5 g fiber
46 g sugar
3 g protein

1 ripe banana

¾ cup frozen mango

½ cup orange juice

½ cup 2% Greek-style yogurt

▼

Combine all ingredients in a blender and puree until smooth.

MAKES 1 SERVING

Sweet Stir-Prize

Stir-frys are naturally high in sodium, but this stir-fry flips the tables by wedding potassium powerhouses like sweet potatoes and broccoli with juicy chunks of chicken and a spicy-sweet sauce built with orange juice and chili sauce. Make it the night before and pack it up for a perfect office lunch.

▼

Stir together the soy sauce, Sriracha, orange juice, vinegar, and cornstarch in a small mixing bowl. Set aside.

Heat half the oil in a wok or large stainless steel pan over high heat. Add the chicken, stirring occasionally with a spatula or metal spoon, and cook until browned all over, about 3 minutes total. Remove to a plate and reserve.

Turn the heat down to medium and add the remaining oil. Add the sweet potatoes, broccoli, onions, garlic, and ginger. Cook, stirring occasionally, until the vegetables have softened, about 8 minutes. Add the soy-orange juice mixture to the pan along with the chicken, toss to coat.

Serve with steamed brown rice.

MAKES 4 SERVINGS

240 calories / 8 g fat / 2 g sat fat /
410 mg sodium / 4 g fiber / 3 g sugar / 25 g protein

2 Tbsp low-sodium soy sauce

½ Tbsp Sriracha, or other Asian-style chili sauce

2 Tbsp orange juice

1 Tbsp rice wine vinegar

½ Tbsp cornstarch

1 Tbsp peanut or canola oil

1 lb boneless skinless chicken thighs, cut into bite-size pieces

1 medium sweet potato, peeled and sliced into thin rounds

4 cups broccoli florets

1 small yellow onion, sliced

2 cloves chopped garlic

1 Tbsp fresh minced ginger

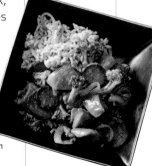

200 calories
5 g fat
1 g sat fat
115 mg sodium
3 g fiber
3 g sugar
24 g protein

DINNER

HALIBUT A LA UPS

Among the cocktail of nutrients that can help improve blood pressure, halibut boasts impressive reserves of three of the most important: potassium, magnesium, and omega-3 fatty acids. Here it's combined with other blood-pressure beaters like fennel and mushrooms in the kind of dead-simple technique that will make you look like a culinary genius. Simply wrap the halibut up with the other ingredients (feel free to improvise, too) in parchment paper, place in the oven, and take it straight to the plate. The best part? No cleanup.

▼

Preheat oven to 450°F.

Lay out the sheets of parchment paper (or aluminum foil) on a flat work surface. Place a piece of fish in the center of each sheet, drizzle with a bit of olive oil, and season with salt on both sides. Top with a lemon slice and equal portions of the tomatoes, fennel, mushrooms, and garlic. Season the vegetables with salt and black pepper.

Just before sealing the packets, add 2 tablespoons of white wine to each packet. To seal the packets, fold the paper or foil over the fish and roll up the edges to create a tight pouch. Place on a baking sheet and cook in the oven for 12 to 15 minutes, depending on how thick the fish is.

MAKES 4 SERVINGS

4 pieces parchment paper or large pieces of aluminum foil

1 lb halibut (other firm white fish such as swordfish or mahi mahi will work as well)

1 Tbsp olive oil

Salt and black pepper to taste

4 thin slices lemon

1 pint cherry tomatoes

1 bulb fennel, thinly sliced

8 cremini mushroom caps, stemmed and halved

2 cloves garlic, minced

½ cup white wine

COOK IT TO BEAT IT!

BEAT DIABETES

BEAT IT!

A key component to preventing diabetes is avoiding too much of a good thing—in this case, blood sugar, otherwise known as glucose, the stuff that feeds your brain and powers your body, until you get too much of it. Over time, as high-calorie, high-sugar foods spike your blood glucose levels over and over again, your body's insulin receptors become worn down (insulin is the hormone that helps keep blood sugar stable). So the key to dodging the diabetes bullet is to focus on foods that are low in sugar and high in protein and fiber (both of which are digested slowly and keep your blood sugar levels stable). These meals are loaded with both. Those who eat the least fiber (20 grams or less a day) have the greatest chance of getting diabetes, according to a recent study in the journal *Diabetes Care*.

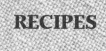

The
Bossest
Sausage

Forgive Us Our Cinnamon Oatmeal

Sure, you can do instant oatmeal, but Quaker's version of this bowl contains 12 ingredients, half of which you won't recognize as food. The scratch-made version is gentle on your blood sugar, containing the soluble fiber of the oats and two of the secret weapons of the diabetic's pantry: cinnamon, shown in countless studies to help regulate insulin levels, and agave syrup, a sweetener that tastes just like sugar but doesn't affect your blood sugar.

1 cup water
½ cup quick-cooking oats
1 cup diced Granny Smith apple
Pinch salt
½ tsp cinnamon
1 Tbsp agave syrup

▼

Bring the water to a boil. Stir in the oatmeal and apples and season with a pinch of salt. Cook until the oats are soft, about 2 to 3 minutes. Stir in the cinnamon and the agave syrup and serve.

MAKES 1 SERVING

450 calories
1.5 g fat
0 g sat fat
410 mg sodium
7 g fiber
28 g sugar
11 g protein

BIRDS IN THE TREES

Sweet, tender leaves of lettuce play the role of delivery system here—a trick taken from Asian cuisines that mastered the art of low-calorie wraps long ago.* Not only is this is a high-protein, low-carb lunch, but it has at its core a potent diabetes defender. Curcumin, a compound in turmeric, a major component of curry powder, was found in a recent Thai study to help prevent the onset of diabetes in pre-diabetics. The fact that curry goes beautifully in chicken salad—especially one laced with the sweetness of carrots and golden raisins—is all the more reason to quadruple this recipe and keep it in your fridge all week.

▼

In a small mixing bowl, combine the chicken, carrot, celery, raisins, mayonnaise, vinegar, and curry powder. Season to taste with salt and pepper. Serve by scooping a big spoonful of the salad onto a lettuce leaf and eating.

MAKES 1 SERVING

*Of course, if you want this on bread, no problem—try low-carb, low-calorie Sandwich Thins, made by both Arnold and Oroweat.

1 cup cooked chicken (grilled chicken breast, leftover roast chicken, or a store-bought rotisserie bird all work perfectly)

¼ cup grated carrot

1 stalk celery, diced

1 Tbsp golden raisins

2 Tbsp olive oil–based mayonnaise

1 tsp white wine or apple cider vinegar

1 tsp curry powder

Salt and black pepper to taste

4 large leaves Boston or Bibb lettuce

500 calories / 28 g fat / 4.5 g sat fat / 360 mg sodium / 4 g fiber / 8 g sugar / 46 g protein

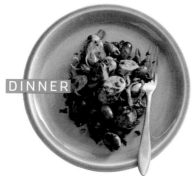

DINNER

The Bossest Sausage

Hot grapes and sausage may sound like an unlikely pair, but one bite of the sweet-savory combination and you'll be convinced. Not only is the meal low in carbs and high in protein and fiber (thanks, kale!), but research has connected red grape consumption to better blood sugar balance and insulin regulation.

- 1 tsp olive oil
- 4 links uncooked chicken sausage
- 1 medium red onion, sliced
- 2 cloves garlic, thinly sliced
- 2 cups red grapes
- 1 tsp fennel seeds
- 2 cups chopped kale
- 2 Tbsp red wine or balsamic vinegar
- Salt and black pepper to taste

Heat the olive oil in a large cast-iron skillet or stainless steel pan over medium heat. Add the sausages and onion and cook until the meat is nicely browned on one side, about 4 minutes. Flip and add the garlic, grapes, and fennel seeds. Continue cooking until the sausage is browned on both sides and firm to the touch. Add the kale and the vinegar. Cook until the kale is soft and wilted, about 2 minutes more. Season with salt and black pepper to taste.

MAKES 4 SERVINGS

270 calories
11 g fat
2 g sat fat
700 mg sodium
2 g fiber
13 g sugar
25 g protein

THE EAT IT TO BEAT IT! NO-FLY ZONE

CHAPTER 5

I'm not going to tell you not to eat your favorite foods—pizza, wings, burgers, steaks, ice cream, chocolate, you name it. And I'm not going to tell you not to go to your favorite restaurants—McDonald's, Baskin-Robbins, Panera Bread, TGI Friday's, whatever tickles your fancy.

But I am going to ask you to do one thing: to stand with me against the foods that are simply too outrageously bad for us. To say, in the immortal words of the guy in that *Babe* movie, "That'll do, pig."

You see, you and I are the lucky ones. We're educating ourselves about nutrition, and learning that we can eat all our favorite foods and still lose weight, beat back the threat of diabetes and heart disease, and protect ourselves from a host of modern ills. With this book in hand, you can venture into any restaurant or supermarket and know you're spending your money wisely and healthfully for you and your family.

But that's not where our responsibility ends. There are a lot of unsuspecting people out there—especially young people—who have no idea how vulnerable they are. We need to let today's big chain restaurants know that they can't serve us food that has more than an entire day's worth of calories, fat, salt, or, worst of all, trans fats.

And yet, that's just what's happening.

LET'S MAKE A STAND!

Our food isn't getting better, it's getting worse. So I'm asking you to join me in taking a pledge: a pledge not to order any of these restaurant items until the folks behind these recipes manage to bring their fat, salt, calorie, and trans fat counts down to <u>an entire day's worth</u>. That's right, I'm not asking for diet food. I'm just asking for a return to sanity. We shouldn't be sold any food that's more than 1,800 calories—the most that a woman should eat in one day; or more than 65 grams of fat, 2,400 milligrams of sodium, or 2 grams of trans fat. And if you try to sell it to us, we ain't buying.

Some of these foods break one of the boundaries of reason. Some break two or more. But all of them should be avoided, period.

Consider this your No-Fly Zone.

NO-FLY ZONE

RESTAURANT	FOOD ITEM	CALORIES No more than 1,800	FAT No more than 65 g	SODIUM No more than 2,400 mgs	TRANS FAT No more than 2 g
A&W	Cheese Curds, Large		80	2,440	
A&W	Reese's Peanut Butter Fudge Blendrrr (32 oz)		79		
A&W	Large Fries				4.5
A&W	Large Breaded Onion Rings				7
Applebee's	Appetizer Sampler	2,370		6,120	
Applebee's	Oriental Chicken Rollup			3,220	
Applebee's	Applebee's Reuben			5,240	
Applebee's	Oriental Grilled Chicken Salad, regular		81		
Applebee's	Crispy Orange Chicken			2,530	
Applebee's	Chicken Fried Chicken			6,090	
Applebee's	Chicken Fajita Rollup			3,060	
Applebee's	4-Cheese Mac & Cheese, with Honey Pepper Chicken Tenders		92	4,300	
Applebee's	Lemon Shrimp Fettuccine			5,160	
Applebee's	American BLT		95	3,190	
Applebee's	Four-Cheese Grille			2,950	
Applebee's	Clubhouse Grille		68	2,940	
Applebee's	Fried Chicken Salad, regular		76	2,510	
Applebee's	Shrimp Combo Platter			5,200	
Applebee's	Sizzling Skillet Fajitas—shrimp			6,110	
Applebee's	Quesadilla Burger		105		
Applebee's	Chocolate Chip Cookie Sundae		75		
Applebee's	Fiesta Lime Chicken + sides		65		
Applebee's	California Shrimp Salad, regular		66		
Applebee's	Double Crunch Shrimp		71		
Applebee's	Cowboy Burger		74		
Applebee's	Blue Ribbon Brownie		77		
Applebee's	Pecan-Crusted Chicken Salad, regular		78		
Applebee's	Southwest Jalapeño Burger		79		
Applebee's	Bourbon Black & Bleu Burger		90		
Applebee's	Hand-Battered Fish & Chips		108		
Applebee's	New England Fish & Chips		126		
Baja Fresh	Steak Nacho Burrito			3,224	
Baskin-Robbins	Chocolate Chip Cookie Dough Shake, large		72		
Bertucci's	Spaghetti with Meatballs, with Bolognese Sauce	1,880		3,740	

RESTAURANT	FOOD ITEM	CALORIES No more than 1,800	FAT No more than 65 g	SODIUM No more than 2,400 mgs	TRANS FAT No more than 2 g
Bertucci's	Baked Tortellini & Chicken Gratinati		67	4,120	
Bertucci's	Pesto Grilled Salmon		86		
Blimpie's	Meatball Parmigiana, large			3,640	
Blimpie's	Special Vegetarian (Doritos Sub), large			3,540	
Blimpie's	Veggie Supreme, large			3,000	
Blimpie's	Chicken Cheddar Bacon Ranch			3,240	
Bob Evans	Smokehouse Fried Chicken Sandwich			2,833	
Boston Market	Meatloaf, large				3
Boston Market	St. Louis Style BBQ Ribs, ½ rack		74	3,150	
Burger King	BK Ultimate Breakfast Platter		84	2,920	
Carl's Jr.	The Western Bacon Six Dollar Burger			2,440	
Carl's Jr.	Biscuits & Gravy				7
Carrabbas	Calamari Ricardo, regular		157		11
Carrabbas	Sostanza With Shrimp			3,339	
Carvel	Carvelanche M&Ms, large		98		
Carvel	Carvelanche Reese's, large		91		
Carvel	Peanut Butter Cup Sundae Dasher, large		111		
The Cheesecake Factory	Shepherd's Pie (lunch)			3,211	
The Cheesecake Factory	B.B.Q. Pulled Pork Sandwich			2,608	
The Cheesecake Factory	Factory Burrito Grande	1,839		3,776	
The Cheesecake Factory	Stuffed Chicken Tortillas			2,847	
The Cheesecake Factory	Shepherd's Pie			4,209	
The Cheesecake Factory	Sunrise Fiesta Burrito			4,600	
The Cheesecake Factory	Orange Chicken			2,850	
The Cheesecake Factory	Chicken and Biscuits	2260	68	2,866	
The Cheesecake Factory	Spicy Cashew Chicken	1,809		4,450	
The Cheesecake Factory	Teriyaki Chicken			2,793	
The Cheesecake Factory	Pasta Carbonara	2,134			
The Cheesecake Factory	Fettuccini with Chicken and Sun-Dried Tomatoes	1,832			
The Cheesecake Factory	Louisiana Chicken Pasta	2,052			
The Cheesecake Factory	Farfalle with Chicken and Roasted Garlic	2,193			
The Cheesecake Factory	Bistro Shrimp Pasta	2,285			
The Cheesecake Factory	Miso Salmon			2,416	
The Cheesecake Factory	Steak Diane and Chicken Madeira			2,477	

RESTAURANT	FOOD ITEM	CALORIES No more than 1,800	FAT No more than 65 g	SODIUM No more than 2,400 mgs	TRANS FAT No more than 2 g
The Cheesecake Factory	Beef Ribs			2,310	
The Cheesecake Factory	Monte Cristo Sandwich			2,775	
The Cheesecake Factory	French Toast with Bacon	1,849		3,114	
Chili's	Texas Cheese Fries		117	5,270	
Chili's	Bacon Ranch Steak Quesadilla		139		
Chili's	Boneless Buffalo Chicken Salad			4,720	
Chili's	Quesadilla Explosion Salad		96	3,090	
Chili's	Bacon Avocado Chicken Sandwich		76	3,890	
Chili's	Honey-Chipotle Chicken Crispers		77	4,100	
Chili's	Skillet Chocolate Chip Cookie		71		
Cold Stone	Cake n Shake		69		
Cold Stone	Mud Pie Mojo, Gotta Have It		80		
CPK	Italian Deli Sandwich, with Herb Cheese			3,190	
CPK	Full Moroccan Spiced Chicken Salad		99		
CPK	Chicken Milanese		76		
Dairy Queen	Georgia Mud Fudge Blizzard, large		79		
Denny's	Double Cheeseburger				4
Denny's	The Grand Slamwich, with hash browns		102	3,690	4
Denny's	Fish and Chips		73		
Denny's	BBQ Bacon Cheddar Burger with fries		88		
Denny's	Oreo Milk Shake		73		4
Friendly's	Hunka Chunka Pb Fudge Lava Cake Sundae		107		
Friendly's	Giant Crowd Pleaser Sundae	2,390			
Friendly's	Reese's Peanut Butter Cup 5 Scoop		70		
Friendly's	Caramel Fudge Oreo Brownie Sundae		66		
Friendly's	Kickin' Buffalo Chicken Strips		116	3,040	
Friendly's	Loaded Waffle Fries		119	4,830	
Friendly's	Honey BBQ Chicken Supermelt		78	2,410	
IHOP	Mega Monster Cheeseburger				4
IHOP	Fried Chicken Dinner		84	3,980	4
IHOP	Country/Chicken Fried Steak & Eggs, with Sausage Gravy		115	4,550	
IHOP	Crispy Chicken Salad, with Fried Chicken		88	2,770	
IHOP	Chicken Clubhouse Stacker		83	2,750	
Jack in the Box	Sirloin Swiss & Grilled Onion Burger with Bacon		69		

FAT
No more than 65 g

SODIUM
No more than 2,400 mgs

CALORIES
No more than 1,800

TRANS FAT
No more than 2 g

RESTAURANT	FOOD ITEM	CALORIES (No more than 1,800)	FAT (No more than 65 g)	SODIUM (No more than 2,400 mgs)	TRANS FAT (No more than 2 g)
Jake's Wayback	Jake's Wayback Triple Triple Burger		125		
Long Horn	Western Cheese Fries			4,940	
Long Horn	Bananas Foster Cheesecake		98		
Long John Silver's	Breaded Clam Strips snack box				7
Long John Silver's	Battered Onion Rings, 5pc				7
Long John Silver's	Baja Fish Taco				9
Long John Silver's	Fries				4
Nathan's	Nathan's Famous 4:1 Skinless Cheese Dog				3.5
Nathan's	Nathan's Famous 8:1 Natural Casing Cheese Dog				3
Nathan's	Nathan's Famous 6:1 Skinless Cheese Dog				3.5
Nathan's	Chili Cheese Fries		72		
Olive Garden	Chicken & Shrimp Carbonara		88	3,000	
Olive Garden	Tour of Italy		74	3,830	
Olive Garden	Lasagna Classico			2,830	
Olive Garden	Fettuccine Alfredo		75		
Olive Garden	Chicken Alfredo, dinner		82		
Olive Garden	Chicken & Shrimp Carbonara			3,000	
Olive Garden	Seafood Alfredo			2,430	
Olive Garden	Spaghetti with Italian Sausage		67	3,090	
Olive Garden	Chicken Parmigiana			3,380	
Olive Garden	Stuffed Chicken Marsala			2,830	
Olive Garden	Chicken Parmigiana Sandwich, whole			2,580	
Olive Garden	Classic Shrimp Scampi Fritta Sandwich, whole			2,590	
Olive Garden	Spicy Shrimp Scampi Fritta Sandwich, whole			2,750	
On the Border	Grande Taco Salad - Chicken, without Dressing		75		
On the Border	Grande Taco Salad - Ground Beef, without Dressing		85		
On the Border	Firecracker Stuffed Jalapeno, with Original Queso	1,910	135	6,050	
On the Border	New Mexico Border Style Combo		68		
On the Border	Border Sampler	2,060	142	4,110	
On the Border	Baja Border Style Combo		85	2,710	
On the Border	Chicken Salsa Fresca			2,410	
On the Border	Dos XX Fish Tacos, with Creamy Red Chili Sauce	1,950	121	3,540	
On the Border	Southwest Chicken Tacos, with Creamy Red Chili Sauce			2,920	
On the Border	Brisket Tacos, with Jalapeño BBQ Sauce			3,820	

RESTAURANT	FOOD ITEM	CALORIES No more than 1,800	FAT No more than 65 g	SODIUM No more than 2,400 mgs	TRANS FAT No more than 2 g
On the Border	Pork Guajillo Tacos, with Guajillo Steak Sauce			2,410	
On the Border	Superior Dinner		82	3,280	
On the Border	Big Steak Bordurrito, with Side Salad without Dressing		89	3,480	
On the Border	Classic Chimichanga Chicken, without Sauce		79		
On the Border	Classic Chimichanga Ground Beef, without Sauce		90	2,440	
On the Border	Three Sauce Fajita Chicken Burrito			4,540	
On the Border	Three Sauce Fajita Steak Burrito			3,330	
On the Border	Border Brownie Sundae, with Vanilla Ice Cream		72		
On the Border	The Ultimate Fajita		96	2,750	
On the Border	Grilled Enchilada - Pepper Jack Chicken			2,990	
On the Border	Grilled Enchilada - Smoky Beef Brisket			2,510	
On the Border	Ranchiladas		66	3,180	
On the Border	Tres Enchiladas - Cheese & Onion, with Chile con Carne		66	2,820	
On the Border	Tres Enchiladas - Ground Beef, with Chile con Carne			2,510	
On the Border	Lunch Fajita Nachos - Chicken			2,850	
On the Border	Dos XX Fish Tacos lunch		82	2,610	
On the Border	Brisket Tacos lunch			2,800	
Outback Steakhouse	Chocolate Thunder from Down Under		105		
Outback Steakhouse	Aged Cheddar Bacon Burger		72		
Outback Steakhouse	Classic Cheeseburger with American Cheese				2.5
Outback Steakhouse	Classic Cheeseburger with Cheddar				2.3
Outback Steakhouse	Classic Cheeseburger with Provolone				2.7
Outback Steakhouse	Classic Cheeseburger with Swiss Cheese				2.7
Outback Steakhouse	Double Burger		73		3.3
Outback Steakhouse	Prime Rib Dip Sandwich			2,850	3
Outback Steakhouse	The Bloomin' Burger		70		3
Outback Steakhouse	The Outbacker Burger				2.3
Outback Steakhouse	New York Strip Steak 14 oz				2.9
Outback Steakhouse	Porterhouse 22 oz		78		4.6
Outback Steakhouse	Ribeye 14 oz				3.9
Outback Steakhouse	Baby Back Ribs, full rack		77		
Outback Steakhouse	Hand-Breaded Chicken Tenders, Buffalo Style				2
Outback Steakhouse	New Zealand Rack of Lamb				2.5
Outback Steakhouse	Aussie Chicken Cobb Salad Crispy, Blue Cheese Dressing		96		2.3

		CALORIES No more than 1,800	FAT No more than 65 g	SODIUM No more than 2,400 mgs	TRANS FAT No more than 2 g
Outback Steakhouse	Aussie Cheese Fries		134		
Outback Steakhouse	Alice Springs Chicken Quesadillas, large		97	3,095	
Outback Steakhouse	Bloomin' Onion		161		
Outback Steakhouse	Wings		163–173		
Panera	Cheese Tortellini with Alfredo Sauce, large			2,430	
Panera	Full Bacon Turkey Bravo on XL Tomato Basil			2,820	
Panera	Full Smokehouse Turkey on Three Cheese hot panini			2,460	
Perkins	Granny's Country Omelette	1,980	78	5,790	
P.F. Chang's	Shrimp with Candied Walnuts		104		
P.F. Chang's	The Great Wall of Chocolate		72		
P.F. Chang's	Philip's Better Lemon Chicken Lunch		88		
P.F. Chang's	Northern Style Spare Ribs			3,070	
P.F. Chang's	Chang's Spare Ribs			3,750	
P.F. Chang's	Egg Drop Soup Bowl			2,880	
P.F. Chang's	Hot & Sour Soup Bowl			7,980	
P.F. Chang's	Wonton Soup Bowl			3,360	
P.F. Chang's	Chang's Chicken Noodle Soup Bowl			2,400	
P.F. Chang's	Mandarin Chicken			2,930	
P.F. Chang's	Almond & Cashew Chicken			3,780	
P.F. Chang's	Chicken with Black Bean Sauce			3,130	
P.F. Chang's	Mongolian Beef			2,700	
P.F. Chang's	Shaking Beef			2,930	
P.F. Chang's	Beef withBroccoli			3,260	
P.F. Chang's	Pepper Steak			3,000	
P.F. Chang's	Kung Pao Shrimp			2,610	
P.F. Chang's	Shrimp, with Lobster Sauce			2,690	
P.F. Chang's	Hunan Style Hot Fish			3,550	
P.F. Chang's	Lemongrass Grilled Norwegian Salmon			3,180	
P.F. Chang's	P.F. Chang's Fried Rice Combo			2,440	
P.F. Chang's	Lo Mein Chicken			3,040	
P.F. Chang's	Lo Mein Beef			3,180	
P.F. Chang's	Lo Mein Pork			3,130	
P.F. Chang's	Lo Mein Shrimp			3,150	
P.F. Chang's	Lo Mein Vegetable			2,870	

NO-FLY ZONE

		CALORIES No more than 1,800	FAT No more than 65 g	SODIUM No more than 2,400 mgs	TRANS FAT No more than 2 g
P.F. Chang's	Lo Mein combo			3,400	
P.F. Chang's	Singapore Street Noodles			2,750	
P.F. Chang's	Pad Thai Chicken			3,720	
P.F. Chang's	Pad Thai Shrimp			3,840	
P.F. Chang's	Pad Thai Combo			3,780	
P.F. Chang's	Dan Dan Noodles			6,190	
P.F. Chang's	Garlic Noodles			2,990	
P.F. Chang's	Buddha's Feast Stir Fried			3,440	
P.F. Chang's	Ma Pa Tofu			3,450	
P.F. Chang's	Stir-Fried Eggplant			3,350	
P.F. Chang's	Spicy Green Beans, large			2,600	
P.F. Chang's	Shanghai Cucumbers, large			2,540	
P.F. Chang's	Egg Drop Soup Bowl lunch			2,880	
P.F. Chang's	Hot & Sour Soup Bowl			7,980	
P.F. Chang's	Wonton Soup Bowl			3,360	
Popeye's	Cajun Fries, Large				3.5
Quiznos	Bourbon Steak LTO, regular			3,130	
Quiznos	Bourbon Steak LTO, large			4,320	.
Quiznos	Black Angus Steak sub, large			3,080	
Quiznos	Roast Beef & Horseradish, large			2,860	
Quiznos	Peppercorn Prime Rib, regular			2,610	
Quiznos	Peppercorn Prime Rib, large		67	3,590	
Quiznos	French Dip, regular			3,180	
Quiznos	French Dip, large		67	4,160	
Quiznos	Double Swiss Prime Rib, regular			2,830	
Quiznos	Double Swiss Prime Rib, large			3,890	
Quiznos	Mesquite Chicken Sub, large			3,260	
Quiznos	Pesto Caesar Chicken Sub, large			2,690	
Quiznos	Baja Chicken Sub, large			3,540	
Quiznos	Carbonara Chicken Sub, large		66	3,340	
Quiznos	Honey Mustard Chicken Sub, large			3,060	
Quiznos	Honey Bourbon Chicken Sub, large			2,550	
Quiznos	Turkey, Ranch & Swiss Sub, large			3,040	
Quiznos	Turkey Bacon Guacamole Sub, regular			2,820	

Restaurant	Item	CALORIES No more than 1,800	FAT No more than 65 g	SODIUM No more than 2,400 mgs	TRANS FAT No more than 2 g
Quiznos	Turkey Bacon Guacamole Sub, large		69	3,870	
Quiznos	Turkey Lite Sub, large			2,680	
Quiznos	Ultimate Club Turkey Sub, regular			2,780	
Quiznos	Ultimate Club Turkey Sub, large			5,820	
Quiznos	Classic Italian Sub, large			3,370	
Quiznos	The Traditional, large			2,890	
Quiznos	Spicey Monterey, large			3,220	
Quiznos	Honey Bacon Club, large			3,400	
Quiznos	Tuna, large			2,740	
Quiznos	Meatball, regular			2,650	
Quiznos	Meatball, large		76	3,560	
Quiznos	Cobb Salad, large		67		
Quiznos	Peppercorn Caeser Salad, large		70		
Quiznos	Broccoli Cheese Soup, large			2,460	
Red Lobster	Spicy Chicken Tortilla Soup, bowl			2,420	
Red Lobster	Seaside Shrimp Trio			3,630	
Red Lobster	Admiral's Feast		70	3,830	
Red Lobster	Ultimate Feast			2,790	
Red Lobster	Parmesan-Crusted Chicken Alfredo		67	2,920	
Red Lobster	Cajun Chicken Linguini Alfredo, full		73	3,370	
Red Lobster	NY Strip and Rock Lobster Tail			2,820	
Red Lobster	Honey BBQ Shrimp and Chicken			2,770	
Red Lobster	Grilled Chicken with Portobello Wine Sauce			2,450	
Red Lobster	Island Grilled Mahi-Mahi and Shrimp			2,420	
Romano's	Parmesan-Crusted Sole		104		
Romano's	Chicken Under a Brick		115	3,640	
Ruby Tuesday	Chicken & Broccoli Pasta		95	2,838	
Ruby Tuesday	Parmesan Chicken Pasta		74	3,481	
Ruby Tuesday	Chicken & Mushroom Alfredo		66	3,401	
Ruby Tuesday	Bacon Cheeseburger, includes fries		79	2,902	
Ruby Tuesday	Classic Cheeseburger, includes fries		74	2,699	
Ruby Tuesday	Ruby's Classic Burger, includes fries		70	2,519	
Ruby Tuesday	Smokehouse Burger, includes fries		86	3,265	
Ruby Tuesday	Triple Prime Bacon Cheddar Burger, includes fries		91	2,586	

NO-FLY ZONE

		CALORIES No more than 1,800	FAT No more than 65 g	SODIUM No more than 2,400 mgs	TRANS FAT No more than 2 g
Ruby Tuesday	Triple Prime Burger, includes fries		74		
Ruby Tuesday	Triple Prime Cheddar Burger, includes fries		86		
Ruby Tuesday	Spicy Jalapeño Pretzel Cheeseburger, includes fries		87	3,212	
Ruby Tuesday	Portabella Crispy Onion Pretzel Cheeseburger, includes fries		89	3,027	
Ruby Tuesday	Black & Blue Bacon Pretzel Burger, includes fries		90	3,647	
Ruby Tuesday	Bacon Cheese Pretzel Burger, includes fries		101	3,660	
Ruby Tuesday	Avocado Turkey Burger, includes fries		71	2,704	
Ruby Tuesday	Buffalo Chicken Burger, includes fries			3,299	
Ruby Tuesday	Chicken BLT, includes fries			3,042	
Ruby Tuesday	Avocado Grilled Chicken Sandwich, includes fries			2,491	
Ruby Tuesday	Turkey Burger, includes fries			2,459	
Ruby Tuesday	Louisiana Fried Shrimp			3,040	
Ruby Tuesday	Black Fire New York Strip Steak			2,473	
Ruby Tuesday	Ribs & Louisiana Fried Shrimp - BBQ			3,405	
Ruby Tuesday	Ribs & Louisiana Fried Shrimp - Memphis			3,135	
Ruby Tuesday	Parmesan Shrimp Pasta			3.840	
Ruby Tuesday	Cajun Jambalaya Pasta			3.715	
Ruby Tuesday	Chicken & Broccoli Pasta		95	2,838	
Ruby Tuesday	Parmesan Chicken Pasta		74	3,481	
Ruby Tuesday	Chicken & Mushroom Alfredo		66	3,401	
Ruby Tuesday	Santa Fe Chicken Quesadilla, includes fries			2,585	
Sbarro	Pepperoni Stromboli, 1 slice			2,600	
Sbarro	Sausage & Pepperoni Stromboli, 1 slice			2,850	
Sbarro	Fish Fillets Frances		123		
Sbarro	Baked Lasagna			2,470	
Sbarro	Fettuccine Alfredo		115	4,160	
Sbarro	Pasta Rustica with Chicken			3,870	
Sbarro	Pasta Rustica without Chicken			4,500	
Sbarro	Spaghetti with Chicken Parmagiana			3,580	
Sbarro	Spaghetti with Eggplant Parmagiana			2,420	
Sbarro	Linguini with Vegetables			2,670	
Sonic	Supersonic Double Cheeseburger with Mayo		81		
Sonic	Supersonic Double Cheeseburger with Ketchup		76		
Sonic	Supersonic Bacon Double Cheeseburger with Mayo		87		

RESTAURANT	FOOD ITEM	CALORIES No more than 1,800	FAT No more than 65 g	SODIUM No more than 2,400 mgs	TRANS FAT No more than 2 g
Sonic	Supersonic Double Cheeseburger With Mustard		76		
Sonic	Supersonic Jalapeño Double Cheeseburger		76		
Sonic	Oreo Sonic Blast, medium		65		
Sonic	Oreo Sonic Blast, large		93		
Sonic	M&M's Sonic Blast, medium		65		
Sonic	M&M's Sonic Blas, large		94		
Sonic	Reese's Peanut Buttercup Sonic Blast, large		83		
Sonic	Butterfinger Sonic Blast, large		92		
Sonic	Snickers Sonic Blast, medium		67		
Sonic	Snickers Sonic Blast, large		97		
Sonic	Hot Fudge Shake, large		74		
Sonic	Hot Fudge Malt, large		68		
Steak 'n Shake	Slinger Skillet—Sausage			2,700	
Steak 'n Shake	7 X 7 Steakburger		98	4,490	3.5
Steak 'n Shake	Veggie Melt with Portobellos				4
Steak 'n Shake	Chili Deluxe, bowl		74	2,560	
Steak 'n Shake	Chili Cheese Fries, large		67		
Steak 'n Shake	Nacho Fries		68	5,250	
Steak 'n Shake	Sausage Gravy & Biscuits				8
TGI Friday's	Crispy Green Bean Fries		65		
TGI Friday's	Loaded Skillet Chip Nachos		100	4,100	
TGI Friday's	Baby Back Ribs, full rack		72	3,150	
TGI Friday's	Baby Back Ribs, ½ rack			2,440	
TGI Friday's	Jack Daniel's Ribs		73	3,220	
TGI Friday's	Sizzling Chicken & Shrimp		78	2,670	
TGI Friday's	Sizzling Chicken & Cheese		70	2,680	
TGI Friday's	Friday's Shrimp			2,870	
TGI Friday's	Crispy Chicken Fingers		66	2,730	
TGI Friday's	Parmesan-Crusted Chicken			2,600	
TGI Friday's	Hibachi Chicken Skewers			4,760	
TGI Friday's	Hibachi Steak Skewers			3,840	
TGI Friday's	Spicy Craft Beer–Cheese Burger		84	2,540	
TGI Friday's	Steakhouse Bleu Cheese Burger		85	3,290	
TGI Friday's	Jack Daniel's Burger		73	3,500	2

RESTAURANT	FOOD ITEM	CALORIES No more than 1,800	FAT No more than 65 g	SODIUM No more than 2,400 mgs	TRANS FAT No more than 2 g
TGI Friday's	Sedona Black Bean Burger		71	3,400	
TGI Friday's	Turkey Burger			2,570	
TGI Friday's	Cheeseburger		71	2,940	
TGI Friday's	New York Cheddar & Bacon Burger		88	3,880	2
TGI Friday's	Jack Daniel's Chicken Sandwich			3,140	
TGI Friday's	Pecan-Crusted Chicken Salad		102		
TGI Friday's	Tennessee BBQ Pulled Pork Sandwich			3,060	
TGI Friday's	Triple Stack Reuben			3,110	
TGI Friday's	Jack Daniel's Black Angus Rib-Eye & Grilled Shrimp Scampi			5,930	
TGI Friday's	Jack Daniel's Black Angus Rib-Eye			4,510	
TGI Friday's	Jack Daniel's Salmon			4,140	
TGI Friday's	Jack Daniel's Salmon & Grilled Shrimp Scampi			5,560	
TGI Friday's	Jack Daniel's Ribs and Shrimp		80	4,140	
TGI Friday's	Jack Daniel's Ribs		73	3,220	
TGI Friday's	Jack Daniel's Flat Iron			2,550	
TGI Friday's	Jack Daniel's Sirloin & Shrimp			3,480	
TGI Friday's	Jack Daniel's Chicken & Shrimp			2,630	
TGI Friday's	Jack Daniel's Chicken			3,120	
TGI Friday's	Jack Daniel's Black Angus Sirloin & Half-Rack of Ribs			3,780	
Uno Chicago Grill	Super Chi-Town Tasting Plate	2,270	146		
Uno Chicago Grill	Mega Size Deep Dish Sundae	2,700	130		
Uno Chicago Grill	Macaroni and Cheese		134		
Uno Chicago Grill	Fish and Chips		89	3,250	
Uno Chicago Grill	Pizza Skins		140		
Wendy's	¾ lb. Triple with Cheese		66		4
Wendy's	Baconator				2.5
Wendy's	½ lb. Double with Cheese				2.5

THE EAT IT TO BEAT IT! FOOD ADDITIVE GLOSSARY

There are more than 3,000 natural and chemical additives that can be used in our food today, and as you've seen throughout this book, they aren't always things we'd choose to eat if we knew exactly what they were.

To help you understand a bit better the food labels you'll encounter in your quest for better health, I've put together this glossary that describes and analyzes the most common food additives in the aisles, from the nutritious (inulin) to the downright frightening (interesterified fat).

Acesulfame Potassium (Acesulfame-K)

A calorie-free artificial sweetener 200 times sweeter than sugar. It is often used with other artificial sweeteners to mask a bitter aftertaste.

FOUND IN: More than 5,000 food products worldwide, including diet soft drinks and no-sugar-added ice cream.

WHAT YOU NEED TO KNOW: Although the FDA has approved it for use in most foods, animal studies have linked the chemical to lung and breast tumors and thyroid problems.

Alpha-Tocopherol

The form of vitamin E most commonly added to foods and most readily absorbed and stored in the body. It is an essential nutrient that helps prevent oxidative damage to the cells and plays a crucial role in cell communication, skin health, and disease prevention.

FOUND IN: Meats, foods with added fats, and foods that boast vitamin E health claims.

Also occurs naturally in seeds, nuts, leafy vegetables, and vegetable oils.

WHAT YOU NEED TO KNOW: In the amount added to foods, tocopherols pose no apparent health risks, but highly concentrated supplements might bring on toxicity symptoms such as cramps, weakness, and double vision.

Artificial Flavoring

Denotes any of hundreds of allowable chemicals such as butyl alcohol, isobutyric acid, and phenylacetaldehyde dimethyl acetal. The exact chemicals used in flavoring are the proprietary information of food processors, used to imitate specific fruits, butter, spices, and so on.

FOUND IN: Thousands of highly processed foods such as cereals, fruit snacks, beverages, and cookies.

WHAT YOU NEED TO KNOW: The FDA has approved every item on the list of allowable chemicals, but because they are permitted to hide behind a blanket term, there is no way for consumers to pinpoint the cause of a reaction they might have had.

Ascorbic Acid
The chemical name for the water-soluble vitamin C.

FOUND IN: Juices and fruit products, meats, cereals, and other foods with vitamin C health claims.

WHAT YOU NEED TO KNOW: Although vitamin C is associated with no known risks, it is often added to junk foods to make them appear healthy.

Aspartame
A near-zero-calorie artificial sweetener made by combining two amino acids with methanol. Most commonly used in diet soda, aspartame is 180 times sweeter than sugar.

FOUND IN: More than 6,000 grocery items including diet sodas, yogurts, and the tabletop sweeteners NutraSweet and Equal.

WHAT YOU NEED TO KNOW: Over the past 30 years, the FDA has received thousands of consumer complaints due mostly to neurological symptoms such as headaches, dizziness, memory loss, and, in rare cases, epileptic seizures. Many studies have shown aspartame to be completely harmless, while others indicate that the additive might be responsible for a range of cancers.

Azodicarbonamide
A chemical compound in the form of a yellow or orangey red, odorless, crystalline powder, used as a bleaching agent or dough conditioner.

FOUND IN: Cereal, flour, and bread

WHAT YOU NEED TO KNOW: It is primarily used as a blowing agent to make foamed plastics and as an additive in synthetic leather. It's also used to make window and door gaskets, padded floor mats, gym/exercise mats, and shoe soles. It's banned in the UK and Australia.

BHA and BHT (Butylated HydroxyAnisole and Butylated Hydroxytoluene)
Petroleum-derived antioxidants used to preserve fats and oils.

FOUND IN: Beer, crackers, cereals, butter, and foods with added fats.

WHAT YOU NEED TO KNOW: Of the two, BHA is considered the most dangerous. Studies have shown it to cause cancer in the forestomachs of rats, mice, and hamsters. The Department of Health and Human Services classifies the preservative as "reasonably anticipated to be a human carcinogen."

Blue #1 (Brilliant Blue) and Blue #2 (Indigotine)
Synthetic dyes that can be used alone or combined with other dyes to make different colors.

FOUND IN: Blue, purple, and green foods such as beverages, cereals, candy, and icing.

WHAT YOU NEED TO KNOW: Both dyes have been loosely linked to cancers in animal studies.

Brown Rice Syrup
A natural sweetener about half as sweet as sugar. It is obtained by using enzymes to break down the starches in cooked rice.

FOUND IN: Protein bars and organic and natural foods.

WHAT YOU NEED TO KNOW: Brown rice sugar has a lower glycemic index than table sugar, which means it provides an easier ride for your blood sugar. But there have been studies showing that it can contain high levels of arsenic.

FOOD ADDITIVE GLOSSARY

Carrageenan
A thickener, stabilizer, and emulsifier extracted from red seaweed.

FOUND IN: Jellies and jams, ice cream, yogurt, and whipped topping.

WHAT YOU NEED TO KNOW: In animal studies, carrageenan has been shown to cause ulcers, colon inflammation, and digestive cancers. While these results seem limited to degraded carrageenan—a class that has been treated with heat and chemicals—a University of Iowa study concluded that even undegraded carrageenan could become degraded in the human digestive system.

Casein
A milk protein used to thicken and whiten foods and appearing often by the names sodium caseinate or calcium caseinate. It is a good source of amino acids.

FOUND IN: Protein bars and shakes, sherbet, ice cream, and other frozen desserts.

WHAT YOU NEED TO KNOW: Although casein is a by-product of milk, the FDA allows it and its derivatives—sodium calcium caseinates—to be used in "nondairy" and "dairy-free" creamers. Most lactose intolerants can handle casein, but those with broader milk allergies might experience reactions.

Cochineal Extract or Carmine
A pigment extracted from the dried eggs and bodies of the female *Dactylopius coccus,* a beetlelike insect that preys on cactus plants. It is added to food for its dark-crimson color.

FOUND IN: Artificial crabmeat, fruit juices, frozen-fruit snacks, candy, and yogurt.

WHAT YOU NEED TO KNOW: Carmine is the refined coloring, while cochineal extract is comprised of about 90 percent insect-body fragments. Although the FDA receives fewer than one adverse-reaction report per year, some organizations are asking for a mandatory warning label to accompany cochineal-colored foods. Vegetarians, they say, should be forewarned about the insect juices.

Corn Syrup
A liquid sweetener and food thickener made by allowing enzymes to break corn starches into smaller sugars. USDA subsidies to the corn industry make it cheap and abundant, placing it among the most ubiquitous ingredients in grocery food products.

FOUND IN: Every imaginable food category including bread, soup, sauces, frozen dinners, and frozen treats.

WHAT YOU NEED TO KNOW: Corn syrup provides no nutritional value other than calories. In moderation, it poses no specific threat, other than an expanded waistline.

DATEM
Diacetyl tartaric and fatty acid esters of mono and diglycerides (DATEM) is an emulsifyer that is derived from fats from soy, palm, or conala oil, some fruits, and even animal sources. It helps mix fats, oils, and water so they do not separate.

FOUND IN: It's used as a dough strengthener in breads and a foaming agent in spreads and ice creams. It's also used in baked goods, chocolate, chewing gum, and beverages to keep ingredients from separating.

WHAT YOU NEED TO KNOW: When mixed with yeast, DATEM produces MCPDs (monochloropropanediol isomers), which studies have found to cause cancer in animals.

Dextrose
A corn-derived caloric sweetener. Like corn syrup, dextrose contributes to the American

habit of more than 200 calories of corn sweeteners per day.

FOUND IN: Bread, cookies, and crackers.

WHAT YOU NEED TO KNOW: As with other sugars, dextrose is safe in moderate amounts.

Erythorbic Acid

A compound similar to ascorbic acid but with no apparent nutritional value of its own. It is added to nitrite-containing meats to disrupt the formation of cancer-causing nitrosamines.

FOUND IN: Deli meats, hot dogs, and sausages.

WHAT YOU NEED TO KNOW: Erythorbic acid poses no risks, and like ascorbic acid, might actually improve the body's ability to absorb iron.

Evaporated Cane Juice

A sweetener derived from sugarcane, the same plant used to make refined table sugar. It's also known as crystallized cane juice, cane juice, or cane sugar. Because it's subject to less processing than table sugar, evaporated cane juice retains slightly more nutrients from the grassy cane sugar.

FOUND IN: Yogurt, soy milk, protein bars, granola, cereals, chicken sausages, and other natural or organic foods.

WHAT YOU NEED TO KNOW: Although pristine sugars are often used to replace ordinary sugars in "healthier" foods, the actual nutritional difference between the sugars is minuscule. Both should be consumed in moderation.

Fully Hydrogenated Vegetable Oil

Extremely hard, waxlike fat made by forcing as much hydrogen as possible onto the carbon backbone of fat molecules. To obtain a manageable consistency, food manufacturers will often blend the hard fat with unhydrogenated liquid fats, the result of which is called interesterified fat.

FOUND IN: Baked goods, doughnuts, frozen meals, and tub margarine.

WHAT YOU NEED TO KNOW: In theory, fully hydrogenated oils, as opposed to partially hydrogenated oils, should contain zero trans fat. In practice, however, the process of hydrogenation isn't completely perfect, which means that some trans fat will inevitably occur in small amounts, as will an increased concentration of saturated fat.

Guar Gum

A thickening, emulsifying, and stabilizing agent made from ground guar beans. The legume, also known as a cluster bean, is of Indian origin but small amounts are grown domestically.

FOUND IN: Pastry fillings, ice cream, and sauces.

WHAT YOU NEED TO KNOW: Guar gum is a good source of soluble fiber and might even improve insulin sensitivity. One Italian study suggested that partially hydrolyzed guar gum might have probiotic properties that make it useful in treating patients with irritable bowel syndrome.

High-Fructose Corn Syrup (HFCS)

A corn-derived sweetener representing more than 40 percent of all caloric sweeteners in the supermarket. In 2005, there were 59 pounds produced per capita. The liquid sweetener is created by a complex process that involves breaking down cornstarch with enzymes, and the result is a roughly 50/50 mix of fructose and glucose.

FOUND IN: Although about two-thirds of the HFCS consumed in the United States are in beverages, it can be found in every grocery aisle in products such as ice cream, chips, cookies, cereals, bread, ketchup, jam, canned fruits, yogurt, barbecue sauce, frozen dinners, and so on.

WHAT YOU NEED TO KNOW: Since around 1980, the U.S. obesity rate has risen proportionately to the increase in HFCS, and Americans are now consuming at least 200 calories of the sweetener each day. Some researchers argue that the body metabolizes HFCS differently, making it easier to store as fat, but this theory has not been proven.

Hydrogenated Vegetable Oil: See Fully Hydrogenated-Vegetable Oil.

Hydrolyzed Vegetable Protein

A flavor enhancer created when heat and chemicals are used to break down vegetables—most often soy—into their component amino acids. It allows food processors to achieve stronger flavors from fewer ingredients.

FOUND IN: Canned soups and chili, frozen dinners, beef- and chicken-flavored products.

WHAT YOU NEED TO KNOW: One effect of hydrolyzing proteins is the creation of MSG, or monosodium glutamate. When MSG in food is the result of hydrolyzed protein, the FDA does not require it to be listed on the packaging.

Interesterified Fat

A semi-soft fat created by chemically blending fully hydrogenated and nonhydrogenated oils. It was developed in response to the public demand for an alternative to trans fats.

FOUND IN: Pastries, pies, margarine, frozen dinners, and canned soups.

WHAT YOU NEED TO KNOW: Testing on these fats has not been extensive, but the early evidence doesn't look promising. A study by Malaysian researchers showed a 4-week diet of 12 percent interesterified fats increased the ratio of LDL to HDL cholesterol. Furthermore, this study showed an increase in blood glucose levels and a decrease in insulin response.

Inulin

Naturally occurring plant fiber in fruits and vegetables that is added to foods to boost the fiber or replace the fatlike mouthfeel in low-fat foods. Most of the inulin in the food supply is extracted from chicory root or synthesized from sucrose.

FOUND IN: Smoothies, meal-replacement bars, and processed foods trying to gain legitimacy among healthy eaters.

WHAT YOU NEED TO KNOW: Like other fibers, inulin can help stabilize blood sugar, improve bowel functions, and help the body absorb nutrients such as calcium and iron.

L-Cysteine

An amino acid used as a dough stengthener and flavor enhancer.

FOUND IN: Bread and baked goods, sometimes spelled out, sometimes hidden in the bulk term "dough conditioners," and things that call for "meat flavor," like packaged frozen dinners and lunches.

WHAT YOU NEED TO KNOW: It is most often derived from duck feathers and human hair. It is generally recognized as safe by the FDA, and does not always have to appear on the label.

Lecithin

A naturally occurring emulsifier and antioxidant that retards the rancidity of fats. The two major sources for lecithin as an additive are egg yolks and soybeans.

FOUND IN: Pastries, ice cream, and margarine.

WHAT YOU NEED TO KNOW: Lecithin is an excellent source of choline and inositol, compounds that help cells and nerves communicate and play a role in breaking down fats and cholesterol.

Maltodextrin

A caloric sweetener and flavor enhancer made from rice, potatoes, or, more commonly, cornstarch. Through treatment with enzymes and acids, it can be converted into a fiber and thickening agent.

FOUND IN: Canned fruit, instant pudding, sauces, dressings, and chocolates.

WHAT YOU NEED TO KNOW: Like other sugars, maltodextrin has the potential to raise blood glucose and insulin levels.

Maltose (Malt Sugar)

A caloric sweetener about a third as sweet as honey. It occurs naturally in some grains, but as an additive it is usually derived from corn. Food processors like it because it prolongs shelf life and inhibits bacterial growth.

FOUND IN: Cereal grains, nuts and seeds, sports beverages, deli meats, and poultry products.

WHAT YOU NEED TO KNOW: Maltose poses no threats other than those associated with other sugars.

Mannitol

A sugar alcohol that's 70 percent as sweet as sugar. It provides fewer calories and has a less drastic effect on blood sugar.

FOUND IN: Sugar-free candy, low-calorie and diet foods, and chewing gum.

WHAT YOU NEED TO KNOW: Because sugar alcohols are not fully digested, they can cause intestinal discomfort, gas, bloating, flatulence, and diarrhea.

Modified Food Starch

An indefinite term describing a starch that has been manipulated in a nonspecific way. The starches can be derived from corn, wheat, potato, or rice, and they are modified to change their response to heat or cold, improve their texture, and create efficient emulsifiers, among other reasons.

FOUND IN: Most highly processed foods,

low-calorie and diet foods, pastries, cookies, and frozen meals.

WHAT YOU NEED TO KNOW: The starches themselves appear safe, but the nondisclosure of the chemicals used in processing causes some nutritionists to question their effects on health, especially of infants.

Mono- and Diglycerides

Fats added to foods to bind liquids with fats. They occur naturally in foods and constitute about 1 percent of normal food fats.

FOUND IN: Peanut butter, ice cream, margarine, baked goods, and whipped topping.

WHAT YOU NEED TO KNOW: Aside from being a source of fat, the glycerides themselves pose no serious health threats.

Monosodium Glutamate (MSG)

The salt of the amino acid glutamic acid, used to enhance the savory quality of foods. MSG alone has little flavor, and exactly how it enhances other foods is unknown.

FOUND IN: Chili, soup, and foods with chicken or beef flavoring.

WHAT YOU NEED TO KNOW: Studies have shown that MSG injected into mice causes brain-cell damage, but the FDA believes these results are not typical for humans. The FDA receives dozens of reaction complaints each year for nausea, headaches, chest pains, and weakness.

Natural Flavor

According to the FDA, natural flavors are "the essential oil, oleoresin, essence or extractive, protein hydrolysate, distillate, or any product of roasting, heating or enzymolysis, which contains the flavoring constituents derived from a spice, fruit or fruit juice, vegetable or vegetable juice, edible yeast, herb, bark, bud, root, leaf or similar plant material, meat, seafood, poultry, eggs, dairy products, or fermentation products thereof, whose significant function in food is flavoring rather than nutritional." Translation: any chemical flavor concoction that a chemist can think up, as long as the source of the chemical is from a "natural source."

FOUND IN: Almost every kind of packaged and prepared foods.

WHAT YOU NEED TO KNOW: The seemingly harmless, even healthy-sounding, term can hide bizzare conctions dreamed up by "flavorists" in a lab. Things like castoreum, a natural flavor derrived from the sex glands of beavers (located right next to the anal glands, so it can contain anal secretions), but apparently it smells like vanilla so it's used to give some products like ice creams a "natural" vanilla flavor.

Neotame
The newest addition to the FDA-approved artificial sweeteners. It's chemically similar to aspartame and at least 8,000 times sweeter than sugar. It was approved in 2002, and its use is not yet widespread.

FOUND IN: Clabber Girl and Domino Pure D'Lite.

WHAT YOU NEED TO KNOW: Neotame is the second artificial sweetener to be deemed safe by the Center for Science in the Public Interest (the first was sucralose). It's considered more stable than aspartame, and because it's 40 times sweeter, it can be used in much smaller concentrations.

Olestra
A synthetic fat created by pharmaceutical company Procter & Gamble and sold under the name Olean. It has zero-calorie impact and is not absorbed as it passes though the digestive system.

FOUND IN: Light chips and crackers.

WHAT YOU NEED TO KNOW: Olestra can cause diarrhea, intestinal cramps, and flatulence. Studies show that it impairs the body's ability to absorb fat-soluble vitamins and vital carotenoids such as beta-carotene, lycopene, lutein, and zeaxanthin.

Oligofructose: See Inulin.

Partially Hydrogenated Vegetable Oil
A manufactured fat created by forcing hydrogen gas into vegetable fats under extremely high pressure, an unintended effect of which is the creation of trans fatty acids. Food processors like this fat because of its low cost and long shelf life.

FOUND IN: Margarine, pastries, frozen foods, cakes, cookies, crackers, soups, and nondairy creamers.

WHAT YOU NEED TO KNOW: Trans fat has been shown to contribute to heart disease more so than saturated fats. While most health organizations recommend keeping trans-fat consumption as low as possible, a loophole in the FDA's labeling requirements allows processors to add as much as 0.49 grams per serving and still claim zero in their nutrition facts. Progressive jurisdictions such as New York City, California, and Boston have approved legislation to phase trans fat out of restaurants, and pressure from watchdog groups might eventually lead to a full ban on the dangerous oil.

Pectin
A carbohydrate that occurs naturally in many fruits and vegetables and is used to thicken and stabilize foods.

FOUND IN: Jellies and jams, sauces, pie filling, smoothies, and shakes.

WHAT YOU NEED TO KNOW: Pectin is a source

of dietary fiber and might help to lower cholesterol.

Polysorbates

A class of chemicals usually derived from animal fats and used primarily as emulsifiers, much like mono- and diglycerides.

FOUND IN: Cakes, icing, bread mixes, condiments, ice cream, and pickles.

WHAT YOU NEED TO KNOW: Polysorbates allow otherwise fat-soluble vitamins to be dissolved in water, an odd trait that seems to have a benign effect. Watchdog groups have deemed the additive safe for consumption.

Propylene Glycol

A preservative, thickening agent, and stabelizer, used to absorb extra water and maintain moisture content.

FOUND IN: Ice cream, yogurt, salad dressings, candy, and cheese

WHAT YOU NEED TO KNOW: While propylene glycol is generally recognized as safe by the USDA, it is also used as antifreeze, and to de-ice airplanes. It is found in electronic cigarettes and used as a plasticizer to make polyester resins.

Propyl Gallate

An antioxidant used often in conjunction with BHA and BHT to retard the rancidity of fats.

FOUND IN: Mayonnaise, margarine, oils, dried meats, pork sausage, and other fatty foods.

WHAT YOU NEED TO KNOW: Rat studies in the early 1980s linked propyl gallate to brain cancer. Although these studies don't provide sound evidence, it is advisable to avoid this chemical when possible.

Red #3 (Erythrosine) and Red #40 (Allura Red)

Food dyes that are orange-red and cherry red, respectively. Red #40 is the most widely used food dye in America.

FOUND IN: Fruit cocktail, candy, chocolate cake, cereals, beverages, pastries, maraschino cherries, and fruit snacks.

WHAT YOU NEED TO KNOW: The FDA has proposed a ban on Red #3 in the past, but so far the agency has been unsuccessful in implementing it. After the dye was inextricably linked to thyroid tumors in rat studies, the FDA managed to have the lake (or liquid) form of the dye removed from external drugs and cosmetics.

Saccharin

An artificial sweetener 300 to 500 times sweeter than sugar. Discovered in 1879, it's the oldest of the five FDA-approved artificial sweeteners.

FOUND IN: Diet foods, chewing gum, toothpaste, beverages, sugar-free candy, and Sweet 'N Low.

WHAT YOU NEED TO KNOW: Rat studies in the early 1970s showed saccharin to cause bladder cancer, and the FDA, reacting to these studies, enacted a mandatory warning label to be printed on every saccharin-containing product. The label was removed after 20 years, but the question over saccharin's safety was never resolved. More recent studies show that rats on saccharin-rich diets gain more weight than those on high-sugar diets.

Sodium Ascorbate: See Ascorbic Acid.

Sodium Caseinate: See Casein.

Sodium Nitrite and Sodium Nitrate

Preservatives used to prevent bacterial growth and maintain the pinkish color of meats and fish.

FOUND IN: Bacon, sausage, hot dogs, and cured, canned, and packaged meats.